Getting Older Being Here

A Psychologist's Guide to Rehab, Nursing Homes, Dementia, Death, and Aging Well

Ileana Báscuas, PhD, ABPP

All the information contained in this book is educational in nature and provided solely as general information. This information does not constitute medical or psychological advice or prescription. If you or your loved one have a medical condition, consult a physician; for mental health issues, consult a psychologist or other licensed professional. The information provided is not a substitute for professional advice or care. Reading this book does not create a professional relationship with the author nor does the author or publisher accept any responsibility or liability for the use or misuse of the information, including suggested resources and checklists, contained in this book.

The opinions expressed are solely the author's and do not represent the opinions of any other professionals, nursing homes, assisted living facilities, or other organizations the author has been associated with during the past several decades. All examples are composites and have been disguised to protect the privacy of the individuals involved.

Getting Older, Being Here, A Psychologist's Guide to Rehab, Nursing Homes, Dementia, Death, and Aging Well Copyright ©2016 by Ileana Báscuas, PhD, ABPP. All rights reserved.
Printed in USA.

EBook ISBN: 978-0-9971030-0-7
Softbound ISBN: 978-0-9971030-1-4

No part of this publication may be used or reproduced, stored in a retrieval system, transmitted in any form or by any means, electronic, mechanical, photocopying, scanning, recording, or otherwise, without prior written permission of the publisher and author except in the case of "fair use" brief quotations.

www.GettingOlderBeingHere.com

Cover Photo: Bahman Farzad
Cover Design: James, GoOnWrite.com
Interior/formatting: Polgarus Studio

Contents

Introduction: *More than We Can Imagine* 1
    The Journey is Personal – And It's Yours 4
    The Book's Structure and Style 5

Chapter 1 - Good and Bad Happen to Everyone 9
    How We Get to Be Who We Are 10
    Changes Come with Age and Illness 15
    The Cornerstone of Managing Stress 17
    Responding to "Why me?" 21
    Time-Tested Tips 26

Chapter 2 - Patterns & Expectations in Rehab 29
    It's Not What You Expect 32
    Expectations Will Ruin Your Day 34
    What's Wrong with Perfection? 37
    Explaining the Basics so Rehab Isn't Done "Wrong" 38
    Understanding the Influence of Past Issues 45
    Time-Tested Tips 48

Chapter 3 - Getting Rehab Right 51
    Question #1: "What happened? What brought you into rehab?" 51
    Question #2: "How do you feel physically? Are you hurting? If yes, where? When does it hurt, and when did it start?" 52
    Question #3: "How are you sleeping?" 54
    Question #4: "How's your appetite? How much are you eating?" 54
    Question #5: "How much water are you drinking?" 56
    Question #6: "Do you drink alcohol? Do you take any drugs not prescribed by your doctor? Do you smoke?" 59
    Question #7: "Do you understand what rehab is? Tell me what you know." 64

Question #8: "How do you feel emotionally? What's your biggest worry this week?" 64
Question #9: "Do you wish you were dead? Are you feeling suicidal?" 67
Time-Tested Tips 71

Chapter 4 - The Rehab Roller-coaster 75
Confronting "What's the Use?" Thinking 76
Handling the Ups and Downs 78
Doing Rehab "Right" 80
Turtle Time 83
Leaving "AMA" 84
"When Do I Get Out of Here?" 86
You Can't Make Someone Happy 88
Going Home 89
• Mistake #1: Doing too much, too fast, too soon. 91
• Mistake #2: Doing too little. 93
Time-Tested Tips 95

Chapter 5 - What Would You Do? 97
The Drill Sergeant 97
The Meddlers 98
Effective Advocates 100
Denial of Mental Health Evaluations & Services 113
The Thin Veil of Racism 115
"What Would You Do?" 119
Time-Tested Tips 126

Chapter 6 - Making and Accepting Hard Choices 129
Kindness When You Least Expect It 130
Responding to "Why Can't I Go Home?" 132
How to Make a Viable, Conscious Decision 138
Time-Tested Tips 150

Chapter 7 - Reframing the Nursing Home Experience ... 153
  Anywhere You Hang Your Hat ... 154
  A Warehouse is Not a Home ... 161
  Choosing a Nursing Home ... 164
  Complaints, Complaints, and More Complaints ... 171
  Roommates, Food, Laundry, and Activities ... 182
  Loss of Freedom and Control ... 187
  Time-Tested Tips ... 189

Chapter 8 - From Depression to New Ways of Being ... 193
  The Capacity for Consent ... 194
  The Need for Touch ... 197
  "Nobody Cares" ... 199
  Depression ... 202
  When a Second Opinion is Warranted ... 206
  The Past is the Present ... 208
  Family Challenges ... 211
  Compassion ... 219
  Time-Tested Tips ... 222

Chapter 9 - The Alzheimer's & Dementia Quagmire ... 223
  "Are they crazy or what?" ... 226
  A Dementia Diagnosis, and the Stages ... 231
  Normal Cognitive Aging ... 237
  Stress Management ... 239
  Dementia & Long-term Care: Top Mistakes ... 241
  "Personality Changes" Caused by Dementia ... 247
  The "Eternal Now" of Dementia ... 249
  "Are We Doomed to Get Alzheimer's?" ... 251
  Time-Tested Tips ... 253

Chapter 10 - Healing in Dying ... 255
  Prolonging Life or Prolonging Death ... 257
  Reasonable Quality of Life ... 261
  Healing in Dying ... 265
  Regrets of the Dying ... 270

Nearing Death 274
Near Death Experiences 277
NDE Qualities.. 279
Moving Forward 282
Grief 284
Time-Tested Tips 287

Chapter 11 - Healthy Aging 289
The Golden Years or the Rusty Years?.............................290
What We Can Do... 292
Gratitude 296
The End is Always a Beginning 298

Appendix 301
Checklists 303
Resources 323

Acknowledgements 331

About the Author 333

Introduction:
More than We Can Imagine

Over twenty years ago, on a sunny Florida morning, I walked into a nursing home for the first time and collided with the staggering suffering old age and infirmity bring. After more than fifteen years in mental health services and having just left a stressful management job, I was intrigued by a position providing psychological services to nursing home residents. Eventually I was offered the job, but I hesitated to take it since I was not a geriatric psychologist (almost none existed at the time). Then again, I had bills to pay and although the job meant less money than I was used to making, the position seemed to be the least nerve-racking option of my choices. I accepted the offer, thinking I would stay in the job for only a year.

Like any good clinician, I immediately began researching this new area to prepare myself. Much to my surprise I found next to no information regarding the psychological assessment and treatment of the very old and deeply sick who resided in a nursing home. I found only a scant amount of research regarding the dementias they exhibited, and no information as to viable treatment options. I also learned that some residents exhibited disruptive behaviors no one understood or had much time and compassion for, but everyone expected the psychologist (me) to fix it.

What in the world was I doing there? What could I possibly offer to help these residents and their families? What could I offer a harried staff, some with little training, some who only did the job for their meager paycheck, and some who had little interest in the emotional health of their patients? And, how would I personally handle the overwhelming pain, sadness, fear, grief, and infirmity that were an everyday reality within these walls?

It didn't take a doctorate in psychology to notice a cry for help existed everywhere I looked, but what to do remained a mystery I couldn't even begin to describe, much less decipher. I spoke to a few colleagues who were somewhat helpful and encouraging, yet they knew as little as I did in this new field. One psychologist, for example, had developed several behavioral programs for common nursing home problems that looked promising. Unfortunately, as I read them I realized none would ever work in a nursing home, and later I found out he'd never worked in a nursing home. For good outcomes, behavioral programs depend on a trained staff to implement the interventions consistently over time and that did not exist, then or even now, in any nursing home I've ever walked into. This is not to say that behavioral interventions are useless or ineffective. As you'll see throughout this book, small, common sense behavioral inventions can make a world of difference in the daily life of a nursing home resident, their families, and the staff.

During those first few days and weeks on my new job I often thought of admitting defeat, walking out the door and going home, or finding an empty bench somewhere and having a good cry. Thankfully, I don't give up easily.

I began talking to the residents, trying to make a connection despite the obvious hurdles. I listened to their stories, as well as their complaints about living in an institution. In the process, I slowly found what made them and their lives unique and meaningful. I also discovered how truly strong the human spirit is in the face of adversity, pain, and the many transitions we travel through in the course of an ordinary life.

Over the next twenty plus years in numerous "skilled nursing homes" and "assisted living facilities" (ALFs) in the State of Florida – from non-profits, to upscale retirement communities

INTRODUCTION

that require hefty entrance fees, to large and small corporate nursing homes – I talked and counseled thousands of residents and their families, and consulted with staff members and medical personnel. I read and attended scores of continuing education seminars, and I learned the State regulations as well as insurance and financial requirements. I explored different ways of tackling the problems and issues that aging, illness, and dying present, and discovered the skills honed in my prior work with children and their families served me now in new and unexpected ways. At times I even veered away from mainstream psychology to find "cutting-edge" approaches or interventions that could help me help someone in pain and ease their suffering. Eventually, I discovered that when life presents us with an overwhelming and unexpected crisis, we must look outside our "box" to find a larger perspective, and through that we find a deeper level of peace and understanding.

The residents with whom I've worked ranged in age from twenty to one-hundred-eleven. They were in short-term "rehab" (rehabilitation following a debilitating illness, injury, or surgery) or long-term nursing home care. Or, they lived in an independent, continuing care retirement community, or a semi-independent "assisted living facility" (ALF; also known as "residential care facility," "personal care home," or "retirement home" in different parts of the country). They came from every walk of life imaginable: every socio-economic class, education, work or profession, race and ethnic background; religion (or no spiritual inclination whatsoever); some with military and combat/POW experience (most without); some with limited language skills, or who spoke no English, or who had forgotten their second language; and some so bigoted even the most accepting and open-minded among us would cringe when they voiced their prejudices. They represented a vast array of medical conditions in addition to age-related decline. Many of them had sensory and mental impairment, if not some level of dementia or Alzheimer's.

As the years have gone by, I've had to deal with my own and my husband's health challenges as well as my parents' decline and eventual death. My father spent almost five years in long-term nursing home care, his dementia and precarious health a constant presence for a significant time period in my life. As a result, I've experienced the issues and challenges all of us may face as we age from both the perspective of an aging psychologist as well as the family member responsible for managing a loved one's care and dying.

The purpose of this book is to share what I've observed and learned during the past three decades in nursing homes and ALFs to help you better understand and manage aging and what it brings into our lives. This is important because no one I've ever met, including myself and my family, is ready for the predicaments that arise, and when the challenge faces you or your loved one, it will test you in unexpected ways.

The Journey is Personal – And It's Yours

If you disagree with any of the information presented – good. Use that difference of opinion, uneasiness, outright anger or confusion to spur you on to explore a topic further. Consult with appropriate professionals, attend classes and lectures, read a few books, or surf the internet. Discuss these issues and the information you find with trusted family members, friends, and professionals so you can discover what works for you and your loved one in your unique situation at this moment in time.

In this book I won't bombard you with dozens of research studies that although useful, may have little relevance to what you're dealing with in everyday life. In my experience, research data in and of itself seldom changes someone's attitude or behavior. Instead, we are moved to change and transformation when something touches us deeply, even shaking us up a little.

What in this book will touch or shake you up?

Maybe it will be a story that breaks your heart open?

Or, it could be a suggestion that unlocks the door to greater inner peace.

Perhaps it will be an example that illustrates a different way of approaching a problem and pushes you beyond long-held beliefs and assumptions.

The Book's Structure and Style

In writing this book, I had to choose how to present material that does not easily divide into clear-cut categories. As a result, some of the information may seem out of sequence. However, over time the pieces will fall into place much like a jigsaw puzzle that at first looks overwhelming and illogical.

As you read through this work, you will notice the terms *resident*, *elder*, *senior*, *patient*, and *loved one* are used interchangeably. I realize some of you may not consider your family member (who is now in a facility) to be a "loved one" due to a variety of factors, such as personality traits, alcohol and/or drug addiction, past abusive behaviors, or a falling-out due to unresolved disagreements. That said, I choose to follow convention and use these common labels. Furthermore, depending on where you live, titles or labels for facilities, personnel, documents, practices, and even diagnoses may differ. Simply change the term in your mind to what you know or what is used where you or your loved one lives, and the confusion should be minimal.

We'll begin our journey by delving into a psychological dynamic almost everyone facing a health crisis falls victim to, and that is "Why me?" thinking. This simple question leads to a relentless current of giving-up that undermines rehab, recovery, and general well-being. In understanding "Why me?" thinking, we need to develop a basic awareness of mind-body psychology and how we become who we think we are. This brief section discusses recent mind-body/brain research, and although that may be unappealing to some readers, I urge you to read those few pages to have a better working foundation for subsequent chapters.

The next four chapters focus on rehab. Among other issues, we'll look at what rehab triggers emotionally as well as how to "do rehab right" to optimize recovery and going home successfully. Long-term care is discussed in the following three chapters, including how to handle common problems and adjustment issues.

Please consider that dementia touches many seniors, whether they are living at home, in an assisted living facility, or in a long-term nursing home. Their dementia will affect the lives of their family, friends, staff, and even the greater community. Then again, realize that not all rehab or long-term care residents have dementia. Consequently, the chapter on dementia and Alzheimer's follows the sections devoted to rehab and long-term care.

Next, you will find chapters devoted to end-of-life issues and decision-making, and some of this material will present new and even unconventional points of view. Lastly, we focus on how to age well and reduce the likelihood of cognitive decline and dementia. Chapters end with practical, Time-Tested Tips that can be applied immediately.

In the Appendix, you'll find two Checklists – Rehab and Long-Term Care – to help you navigate the rough waters of aging and healthcare, whether for a loved one or to prepare yourself for surgery and rehab. I developed these checklists during the years I managed my father's hospitalizations, rehab, and long-term care. However, do not use the checklists and Time-Tested Tips without first reading the book because you will miss valuable information that will help you better understand and use the checklists.

INTRODUCTION

Please read this book with an open, curious mind and a gracious, willing heart. Nursing homes are rarely what people expect, much less what they wish to embrace or learn about, and aging is so much more than we can imagine. Yet our lives in the here and now can be enriched and made easier if we're willing to delve into one of life's more difficult passages. My life certainly has, despite the rocky start I experienced one summer so many years ago.

Ileana Báscuas, PhD, ABPP
Sarasota, Florida

>You were born with potential.
>You were born with goodness and trust.
>You were born with ideals and dreams.
>You were born with greatness.
>You were born with wings.
>You are not meant for crawling, so don't.
>You have wings.
>Learn to use them and fly.
>~ Rumi

Chapter 1
Good and Bad Happen to Everyone

"Why me?" asked the sixty-seven-year-old stroke patient, now bedbound in diapers, the simplest task an overwhelming chore she could not manage alone, her life permanently upended by a major stroke. "What did I do to deserve this?" she added slowly, pushing every word out with effort, a tear etching its way down her cheek.

Almost every one of the thousands of residents in nursing homes and assisted living facilities I've spoken with during the past twenty years has expressed this sentiment in one way or another. It sounds reasonable, given the circumstances. It's something we've all heard and even thought whenever life wasn't going our way. *But those simple words represent a major stumbling block to recovering from an illness, helping an infirmed parent or spouse, or even living a satisfying life.*

Usually we just nod if others express this kind of "Why me?" statement. We don't know what to say in return, and hearing the question makes us vaguely anxious and uncomfortable. Perhaps we even inwardly agree, silently asking ourselves, "Why *did* this awful stroke (or any other illness, disease, dementia/ Alzheimer's, or injury) have to happen? Why Mom? She's never done anything to anybody; she was good to us. Why Dad? He worked hard all his life, fought for his country, lost two brothers…and now this? It's not fair."

Most of us are quite unaware that just asking or thinking the question has a toxic effect on the life of our loved one. When people express, "Why me?" it actually reflects the deeper workings of their psychological make-up. Uttering it is not an actual request on their part for medical information regarding why an illness occurred or even what they could have done to avoid it. Instead, "Why me?" is expressing their fundamental experience of the world as well as their way of being in the world, and it significantly influences whether they heal or cope effectively with a major illness and aging.

To help us begin to appreciate how this seemingly simple and innocent expression can point to something deeper and toxic, we need to take a brief journey into the basic mechanics of the human mind. A little knowledge and understanding opens the door to change, as well as kindness and compassion. Nonetheless, if you find this topic uninviting, skip it and go to the next section. You can always return later if you need to.

> There's only one thing harder than accepting this, and that is not accepting it.
> ~ Byron Katie

How We Get to Be Who We Are

At birth we're the most helpless of mammals, and we remain helpless for the longest period of time. Even our brains are underdeveloped when compared to other animals. A passing glance at a newborn reflects this basic truth of our biological nature. Yet, every newborn also shows us the unmistakable power of life, of a future yet unmapped, moving us in ways we cannot explain and quietly touching our heart.

Our physical fragility makes us uniquely vulnerable since we depend on our parents and caretakers for our survival, and this continues for many years. In particular, our parents are the center of our world as our minds and bodies grow and experience this new existence.

Almost any mother will say that every baby is different from the very beginning. Babies not only have different bodies, but also different temperaments or predispositions. Some babies are calm and easily satisfied, whereas others are sickly, restless, or fussy. Some are curious and adventuresome, while others are shy or engage too little with the world, and so on. Research has told us that the growing baby in the womb is already reacting to the world – whether to sounds, mother's emotions or even what Mom ate for dinner – and developing preferences as a result. This points to the obvious fact that we all come into life with different capabilities and predispositions that are further shaped and reinforced by our encounters with the world.

A baby has been likened to a sponge because it takes the world in with little discrimination, its young, immature brain showing a limited amount of nerve connections and very slow brain waves. One line of research has focused on **neural pathways** that develop in our brains as it matures. These pathways can be viewed as a roadmap, and like any map some pathways are relatively minor and seldom used. Others are strongly imprinted and used often, our default route – our "choice" or pattern we revert to with little if any conscious thought or control. Researchers tell us that our everyday experience involves, among other things, a cascade of chemical reactions and increasing neural pathways in our brains. Over time this becomes what we refer to as our *emotions*, *thoughts*, and *reactions*, that inner sense of who and what we are in the world.

Perhaps more importantly, scientists tell us that our **DNA**, our genetic blueprint, is molded, switched on or off, or intensified by outside influences. **Behavioral epigenetics** research has found that our emotions, beliefs, experiences, behaviors, diet, and other environmental influences (such as toxins, traumas, war, famine) can modify or change our genetic blueprint and its expression in our lives. Even more surprising are findings that point to the emotional experiences and "bad habits" of previous generations leaving a "molecular residue" on our genes which later acts as a trigger for depression, anxiety, addiction, and so forth. In short, how we react may be influenced by the experiences of our lineage, ancestors we may never have met or known about. Additionally, this research also shows we can change the instructions to our genes, that we can modify their expression in our lives.

> The implication is that this basic idea we have that we are controlled by our genes is false. It's an idea that turns us into victims. I'm saying we are the creators of our situation. The genes are merely the blueprints. We are the contractors, and we can adjust those blueprints. And we can even rewrite them.
> ~ Bruce Lipton

Another line of research has looked into our **brain waves** (electrical impulses). From birth to eighteen to twenty-four months the baby's brain is in the sleepy *delta* stage. From age two to six or so, the child's brain is primarily in the drowsy *theta* stage, an extremely impressionable and programmable period. Here, the child basically cannot distinguish what is real from unreal, so their inner experience is their reality. Therefore, most of our programming or conditioning occurs before the age of seven with our parents being are our primary influences.

From roughly age six to eight and onward into adolescence, the brain is developing faster *alpha* waves. These are involved in relaxation, watching TV or movies, daydreaming, intuition, and decreased thinking – but also accelerated learning.

As we age further we develop even faster brain waves known as *beta* where we are alert, able to concentrate, focus, plan, as well as analyze pros and cons. *Beta waves, however, can also indicate over-thinking and worry*, disrupting necessary rest and rejuvenation. Adulthood does not mean we don't experience the "younger" brain waves: Each of the five brain wave patterns (with *gamma* being the fifth) serves a valuable purpose throughout our lives, although they can also be out of balance.

Lastly, deep inside our brains lies the **limbic system**, including the tiny but mighty **amygdala**. The limbic system regulates our emotions and instincts, and determines what memories are stored, especially those related to our survival. Briefly, information comes into our brain through our senses and any danger triggers the amygdala into immediate action and it sends out an alarm to other parts of the brain to ensure our survival. In milliseconds, this process results in a *fight, flight or freeze* reaction. This process drains blood from the brain downward so we can act in the name of survival, but this decreases thinking, and doing so frequently stresses our immune functioning and self-healing.

Importantly, once the amygdala has learned a fear pattern, anything that reminds us of the original threatening or traumatic experience sets off an alarm triggering old memories and emotional reactions that override the rational, thinking mind. Consequently, we react to any such reminders irrationally, out of proportion to the current situation. So, for example, we may say or do whatever pops into our mind with little regard as to whether we're right or hurtful, or what may result from our choices and actions.

Let's look at these processes in action to deepen our practical understanding. For instance, say we're shy and sensitive by nature, and as we grew up our parents emphasized economic security and also often criticized us, expecting some kind of perfection we never achieved. In addition, our lineage experienced famine and the accompanying fear of losing everything. Decades later, when our boss criticizes us, we immediately feel nervous, defeated, and worthless. Before we know it, we're in panic mode and obsessing we're going to lose our jobs. We don't stop to ask ourselves whether what the boss said is true or even significant, much less what we can do about it. We just react with panic, frozen in an old pattern that reaches back generations. This type of commonplace scenario helps illustrate the conclusions of cell biologist Bruce Lipton, who says the brain is *perception* (information via our senses, e.g., our boss's words) whereas the mind is *interpretation* ("I'm no good." "'I'll lose my job. How will I survive?'" "He's never satisfied," and so on).

In addition, research has also shown we are more sensitive to negative experiences, often overlooking and dismissing positive experiences. After all, paying attention to the negative could mean our survival, while the positives only feel good for a short period of time. Furthermore, we'll ruminate or chew on the negatives leading to repetitive, "broken record" thinking that freezes us in a jittery web of anxiety, depression, and inaction. Women, in particular, are more prone to ruminate than men, possibly reflecting the underlying instinct to keep children safe while feeling powerless to control external threats. This rumination and repetition is how a pattern or neural pathway becomes increasingly imprinted in our brain/mind.

Research has also shown we are not capable of suppressing or blocking out our unwanted, scary, or painful thoughts and emotions. And if we try, these only get stronger, once again demonstrating the power of our survival oriented responses, (i.e., the amygdala and limbic system).

It used to be thought that once the amygdala was set in a fear-based pattern it was permanent, and we were doomed to experience this pattern over and over again. Now, we know for a fact that the amygdala and its patterns can be re-set with newer therapies and techniques such as meditation and cultivating self-compassion.

Fortunately, the brain has the ability to change, reorganize, and form new neural connections throughout life as well as compensate for injury and disease (a process called *neuroplasticity*). As a result, we are no longer fated to be helpless victims of our inherited predispositions or negative, fear-based experiences and patterns. This is good news; and the latest findings have opened the door even wider to more research and development of effective therapies and techniques.

> Our thoughts are mainly controlled by our subconscious, which is largely formed before the age of six, and you cannot change the subconscious mind by just thinking about it. That's why the power of positive thinking will not work for most people. The subconscious mind is like a tape player. Until you change the tape, it will not change.
> ~ Bruce Lipton

Changes Come with Age and Illness

In the previous section we learned that each of us is a unique and complex bundle of life, full of vibrant energy with countless ongoing chemical reactions, developing an intricate roadmap of neural pathways within different brain wave patterns as we interact with the world around us. We naturally gravitate to what feels good, safe, and loving, and move away from what feels bad, hurtful, threatening, or scary.

This is our survival mechanism at work, reflecting our basic duality of good or bad, love or fear-based. Love is basically anything that feels good and gives us a sense of security, confidence, and expansion where the world is experienced as kind and supportive. Fear is associated with anything we experience as negative or painful that makes us feel insecure, vulnerable, and helpless, our very existence and well-being seemingly at stake.

Our early programming – and also that of our infirmed loved ones – will surface during the chronic stress of physical decline and illness. This will also happen during medical emergencies, injuries, surgeries, rehab, long-term nursing home placement, and of course, death and dying.

As we all know from experience, aging and illness affects an individual's brain/mind as well as their daily functioning. For most people, the most worrisome outcome is dementia, including Alzheimer's disease, since it signifies a loss of independence, self-control, and identity. But as we'll see later, age-related changes in and of themselves are not as dire and irreversible as many believe, and even a genetic predisposition to Alzheimer's can be modified or reduced by lifestyle habits.

These issues and crises will test us, and few of us are prepared for what life sends our way when body and mind become old, sick, weak, and dysfunctional. Additionally, being a medical patient does not come naturally and will confront us with our fears since we are no longer in control of our lives and at the mercy of strangers. *Luckily, if we are aware of the processes operating during these crises, then we have the opportunity to move into new ways of handling the situation instead of letting old emotional patterns, fear, ignorance, and even stubbornness, rule the day.*

Let's continue to deepen our understanding as we learn what we can do in the here and now to counteract negative patterns and effects. Our **first step** is to *become more aware of any old patterns* – and that begins by noticing how we, and our infirmed loved ones, behave and react. No need for us to *do* anything at this time. Just notice, and we will see early programming in action.

For instance, if you're visiting your loved one in a hospital or nursing home, notice how they are handling their illness and incapacitation, starting with being told what to do.

Also notice your own reaction when you are ill or visiting a loved one: What do you feel in your body? Are you tightening up somewhere? Is your breathing constricted and shallow? Is your stomach queasy? Are you feeling any pain or discomfort?

Are you frustrated, angry, guilty, or resentful? Does your anger skyrocket and you lash out at your loved one, telling them everything they need to do right now to get better?

Do you feel antsy and anxious, as if you need to do something *right now* to fix the situation, or else something bad will happen? Do you think it's all up to you, and that your mother, father, or others will criticize you if you don't fix it or please them?

Or, do you feel you can't wait to leave, wanting nothing more to do with the situation and secretly hoping it'll go away or someone else will take care of it?

If any of these thoughts or feelings come up in you, then stop for a second, and just notice what's going on – with them, and with you. And if the situation becomes too uncomfortable, take a time-out to regroup, like athletes and sports teams do routinely. Take a walk, listen to soothing music, read something inspirational, do a self-help technique that works for you, or take a few slow, deep, cleansing breaths.

> By taking just a few extra seconds to stay with a positive experience — even the comfort in a single breath — you'll help turn a passing mental state into lasting neural structure.
> ~ Rick Hanson

Now that you've noticed some old programming, let's turn to a quick and simple practice you can do for yourself as well as your loved one to *help calm a stressed mind-body and open the door to change.* This is **step two**, and one you can use throughout your day to lessen stress.

The Cornerstone of Managing Stress

Want to be able to have a comfortable visit with your father who has Alzheimer's and can't carry on a conversation? Or stay by your mother's bedside in an intensive care unit? Or say goodbye to a beloved aunt or old friend who's dying in hospice care?

Do you need to remain calm while you're lying in a rehab center recuperating from a painful knee replacement and the nurse is late with your pain medication? Or prevent panic from overtaking you because you've had a stroke and can't talk? Or your rehab is going slower than you expected and your frustration and sense of helplessness is growing with every passing minute?

We can use our breath as a quick and easy way to lower our stress levels, relax our minds, bodies, and emotions, and help our bodies rejuvenate – something many of us need when dealing with the infirmed, or with our own aging and associated illnesses or injuries. Using our breath wisely, we can stop a crying jag or the beginning of a panic attack, even freeing ourselves from a *fight, flight or freeze* response.

It's important to remember that our breath is life itself, enlivening our bodies as well as our brains and what we refer to as our minds. On average we take over twenty thousand breaths every single day. Yet as we go through our busy modern lives, we're often stressed, with stress making our breathing constricted and shallow. If we pay attention, we'll notice our breathing is often in the upper part of our chest, our lungs rarely expanding so our belly gets bigger. If we get nervous, anxious, worried or depressed, our breathing becomes even more restricted which leads to more emotional tension in a never-ending, self-defeating cycle.

How can breathing lower stress, stop crying jags, ease grief, and help us rejuvenate?

Think of an emotion as a wave of energy. Like a wave in the ocean, an emotion flows in and rises to a peak, then ebbs, and returns from whence it came. But we usually interfere with this natural process by trying to control our emotions or push them away, and in so doing this resistance stresses our bodies. If we breathe in a particular way, the emotional wave does not overpower us and cause us to tighten up or trigger wave after wave of stressful, "broken-record" thinking and emotions. Instead, the emotional wave just passes by as it was intended to do, and the mind can rest, yet remain alert and aware. This breathing technique will help us handle any stressful situation that comes our way, and begin to quell the stress of "Why me?" thinking when it leaps out of hiding.

If you're like most people, you'll think this breathing technique is too easy to be effective, or you don't want to try it, feeling an inner resistance rise. This is because we're creatures of habit, and we often try to find any excuse not to do something healthy and beneficial for ourselves if it's new and different. Yet various breathing techniques have a long and successful history, whether used for childbirth, pain control, meditation, sports, or reversing high blood pressure. The breathing technique we're going to embark upon right now is a simple and effective practice, backed by research, and it only takes about twenty seconds.

Try it: It can revolutionize your life and health. Yes, *revolutionize*, since we all seem to have forgotten how to breathe naturally and do what our minds and bodies need to remain healthy.

Here are the simple steps to **4 - 4 Breathing**:

- Breathe in slowly and gently to a count of 4. Imagine your breath going all the way down to your belly button.
- Hold it for a moment or two if you can.
- Then purse your lips and exhale slowly to a count of 4. Imagine your breath flowing outward like a soft breeze.
- Repeat at least 3 times in a row.

Less than three repetitions will not accomplish anything since the brain and nervous system need a certain amount of time to get the message and begin the relaxation process. And if you become more relaxed and centered, you'll be able to think and problem-solve more clearly.

This 4 - 4 breathing technique can be done almost anywhere at any time. Like with any positive habit, the more you do it, the more benefit you will reap.

If you're about to get a root canal or a colonoscopy – *breathe*.

Breathe consciously while you're in your car waiting for the light to change and you tense up over rush hour traffic or what you still need to do, your back pain flaring up. *Breathe*.

Try it when you're nearing your mother's nursing home and feeling your inner stress climb. *Breathe*.

Or, if you can't fall asleep, your thoughts going round and round – *breathe*. You can take care of business tomorrow; it'll still be there waiting for you.

Do 4 - 4 breathing often, particularly during stressful times. Make it a part of your daily life and you'll reap the benefits.

Breathe.

Folks with lung conditions can also do this breathing, only more gently and perhaps only to a count of 3. However, at least three repetitions are still necessary. This will lessen the anxiety they feel when they cannot take a breath like they're used to.

Can you teach your elderly, demented, or infirmed parent or loved one in a hospital, nursing home or ALF to do this breathing? Yes, but do not try to push it on them since that may trigger agitation and confusion if they cannot follow or remember what you say, or simply don't like being told what to do.

If this is the case, focus on doing the 4 - 4 breathing yourself, even when you are in their room with them. You needn't make a big deal out of this; it can be subtle, and few, if any, will notice. The practice will calm you, and create a more peaceful, loving atmosphere in the room. That atmosphere will help your loved one more than you realize.

You can also try this variation, again for several repetitions. Remember, one inhale-exhale cycle will not accomplish anything; we're not wired that way.

- Inhale deep (gently, not a big forced breath which tightens the body).
- Exhale slow into a long sigh.

> And when I breathed, my breath was lightning.
> ~ Black Elk

Responding to "Why me?"

Now that we've learned conscious breathing to help ourselves and our loved one, let's return to the dilemma of "Why me?" In essence, "Why me?" is our experience of conditional love.

As we learned previously, when we're young, our parents and the world around us constantly shower us with information. We're helpless to stop the inflow of information and our parents were the center of our world. In addition, with our immature brains, we had little if any awareness or discrimination as to where they stopped and we began, or what was real versus unreal. This is just the human experience in action, not a failure on anyone's part.

For example, a young child cannot know that Mommy is having PMS and that's why she's grumpy and nitpicking. Or that Daddy is worried about money to repair the leaky roof, and that's why he's short-tempered and raises his voice. A young child also cannot know why Mommy or Daddy yell at them, criticizing them for dropping a glass of milk when they did not drop the glass intentionally. (And the young child does not know they have not developed the small muscles of their hands enough to hold a glass properly.)

The result is that the child receives the message that he is "bad" and not good enough. Each similar experience reinforces and imprints this message in their brain/mind. This scenario – or one similar – happens over and over again in every family, to every child.

Consequently, one of the many things we learn early on is that if we're "bad" or do something that appears to make Mommy or Daddy mad or upset, we get reprimanded, rejected, or punished. And if we're "good," we get rewarded with a treat, a smile, a hug, a kind word or praise. However, the growing child will not understand exactly what the rules and expectations are, much less that it's impossible to please everyone all the time, or be more than what they are at any given time in their development.

Instead, the child learns via a haphazard process of pairing information and experiences, all the while trying to figure out what's expected and what will bring love and security, or avoid criticism. After all, we all want to please Mommy and Daddy and get love, and we all want to avoid their anger and rejection. This is also how we learn conditional love and move away from our natural state of unconditional love.

> Reexamine all that you have been told in school, or in
> church, or in any book. Dismiss whatever insults your soul.
> ~ Walt Whitman

Later, this early programming is reinforced by other caretakers and family members, clergy and church, teachers and school, other children, work, and of course, our culture and media, including social media. And if our parents are religiously minded, they'll bring in some version of "God" as the ultimate father figure who sits in judgment and hands out life's rewards and punishments. Hence, if bad things happen to us – like a major illness or setback – we almost instinctively react with, "Why me? What did I *do* to deserve this?"

In short, *we are reverting back to our early childhood programming, where we think we "did" something to cause the "bad" and painful experience or punishment.* Of course, the severity of the programming, and how the programming shows up in everyday life is individual, varying according to the person and their own unique history. Nonetheless, this "Why me?" thinking is so common to all of us – especially when we're sick and in pain – that we should not dismiss it.

Most people who feel and express this "Why me?" do not have an answer or solution. They just feel bad, even ashamed, about themselves and their apparent failure. More importantly, they don't know what to do to begin to correct or transform how they feel and think, so they feel stuck in negative thinking and harmful self-talk. Also, any debilitating medical condition they have contributes to the problem by weakening them physically and making them feel more vulnerable and more emotional. From there it spirals downward into a deepening sense of powerlessness, self-criticism, depression, and finally, giving up. "Why me?" becomes "What's the use?" and later, "I wish I was dead."

It's important to recognize "Why me?" is a rhetorical question that is voiced *in order to make a point* – not to get an actual answer. This is why it is not a question requesting information regarding how to avoid or correct a medical condition. Therefore, we shouldn't answer it with health or medical information since that will not remedy the problem.

When a person begins expressing, "Why me?" they are actually saying, "This shouldn't be happening to me. I don't deserve this." *Which is what they undoubtedly felt and thought when they were small children. By thinking or voicing "Why me?" they are revealing that they don't understand what they could have done that was so horribly wrong or "bad" that they deserved this painful punishment and fate.*

Given this, how should we respond when they express "Why me?"

First, what we should *not* do is try to explain to a sick or elderly patient that "Why me?" is a rhetorical question; that will not resolve their crisis. In many cases they may not be able to follow this reasoning or information. This type of explanation may make also them feel worse because they'll feel criticized and still don't understand what they should do differently.

Here's what I have come to find works best. Feel free to adapt it for your own use with words and reasoning you are comfortable with, but keep to the original meaning and intent. Of course, use as much or as little of the following as you like.

Or, you can read it to your loved one and say it comes from "Dr. B, the psychologist" (as I'm called in the facilities I work in). Before you begin, however, center yourself with a slow, deep inhale and a long exhale.

For most people, I will answer the question of "Why me?" along the following lines.

> *This is a common reaction. Please know that you did nothing "bad" to warrant the illness or your failing health. Sure, any of us could have made better choices in our life, followed a healthier lifestyle, given up some bad habit or addiction, been kinder to ourselves and others, and so on. But can you absolutely know you were so "bad" – such an awful, unredeemable human being – that you deserve an illness like cancer, stroke, Parkinson's, or Alzheimer's?*
>
> *No, of course not. The evidence of our lives does not support this conclusion.*
>
> *As you know, bad things do NOT only happen to "bad" people. If they did, then how do we account for children getting sick and suffering? What have they done to deserve that fate when they didn't have enough time on this earth to do a lot of "bad" things?*

Every day, people who do mostly good – and of course, make mistakes – get sick too, while some criminals, like murderers and rapists, who do truly bad things, enjoy good health for many years. Think too of good Samaritans like Mother Teresa (India) and Father Damien (leprosy colony in Hawaii) who have also gotten sick, suffered, and even died prematurely.

What is happening to you is simply a part of life. It is the nature of having a human body. After all, the human body is temporary and has an expiration date.

We all get sick or injured sometime, and we all make mistakes as well as enjoy successes of one kind or another. And if we don't die young, we all grow old and eventually experience physical deterioration and death. That's the nature of a human life, not a shameful blunder or some cosmic punishment.

At this point, it's best to leave the resident to digest the new and upended life view they've been presented. There is no need for discussion since that will only prompt the mind to come up with justifications for its old beliefs. Usually, I end by saying, "Think about what I've said, and if you want, we can discuss it next time."

Everyone seems to come around rather quickly because when they "sit with it" for a little while, they see and feel the fundamental error of their childhood logic. The issue now before them is how to move forward, one step at a time, one moment to the next. That's the only way to handle life and what it presents to us, especially when dealing with a major illness or injury and its aftermath.

> If I were to say, 'God, why me?' about the bad things,
> then I should have said, 'God, why me?' about the
> good things that happened in my life.
> ~ Arthur Ashe

Time-Tested Tips

- Breathe deeply and slowly, at least three times in a row. Do it often to reap the benefits.

- Reflect on your early programming and patterns. What are the habitual ways you see and think about the world, yourself, and others? What are the habitual ways you react? What are your attitudes about your body, health, illness, and aging?

- Just *notice*. No need to criticize yourself, or blame your parents and their legacy. What is going on is the nature of being human and our early programming. We simply need to learn more about how life works, how to best manage our mind-body psychology, and cultivate an attitude of compassion toward ourselves as well as others.

- Notice what happens when you get stressed. What do you do? What don't you do? Do you forget to be kind with yourself?

- For the first time we are developing truly effective tools to change our old thinking and patterns. As renown cell biologist Dr. Bruce Lipton has said, "The moment you change your perception is the moment you rewrite the chemistry in your body." And with that change in how we view life, we can begin to rewrite our lives, including our health.

- Please resist the urge to tell your needy, demanding, fretful, self-centered, depressed, cranky, stubborn, irritable, critical, or irascible sick parent or spouse or sibling that they're showing their early programming by being needy, demanding, fretful, self-centered, depressed, cranky, stubborn, irritable, critical, or irascible, and they should stop it now (because you cannot stand it another minute). That will not serve them or you.

  Instead, *breathe*...and take a walk, go home, do something kind and nourishing for yourself. Focus on developing a little more patience, kindness, and compassion toward yourself as well as your infirmed loved one. After all, every one of us can use a little more kindness and self-compassion in our lives.

- Please do not tell your infirmed loved one that they're throwing a "pity party" with their "Why me?" statements. You can certainly use what I've written, but avoid using the information about "Why me?" being a rhetorical question. If what I wrote makes sense to you, then show it, live it, and be a role model to others. The information in this book is meant to be a tool, never a weapon.

- Avoid using any new ideas to force your loved one to do what you think they should do or how you think they ought to be. At best, all we can do is present new information or make simple, concrete suggestions from a place of love, compassion, and understanding. The final decision is that of our loved one, and no one else.

- Don't try to teach someone who is sick or forgetful 4 - 4 Breathing. It may confuse and upset them because they cannot understand it or remember to do it.

- Last but not least, *breathe deeply and slowly at least three times in a row.* Do it as often you can. It's that important, and that powerful.

When you own your breath, nobody can steal your peace.
~ Anonymous

Chapter 2
Patterns & Expectations in Rehab

"This is a prison! I want to go home!"

"You can leave anytime you want. There are no guards at the front door," I said to a man I'd never met before as I practiced my 4 - 4 breathing. The calmer and more centered I am, the more authenticity, clarity, and good intentions I can send out with my words.

Joe, a hulking eighty-five-year-old resident new to rehab, glared at me, his mouth tight with anger and defiance. He was stuck in bed from a recent stroke on top of several age-related maladies, and he was refusing physical therapy and his medications. He repeatedly kicked the nurses and aides out of his room, roaring he wanted nothing to do with the lift that was needed to get him out of bed.

"How are you going to get out of bed and go home? I thought you couldn't walk yet," I added, unafraid of his anger. Though the years I've learned that anger is just an emotion that comes and goes; and there was nothing Joe could do to me except yell and cuss.

"Call my wife! She'll help me!" he blustered.

"Your wife is eighty-three years old, petite, and has to use a walker right now since she's still recovering from her broken hip. How is she going to get you out of bed, help you go to the bathroom, shower and dress, or change your diapers? How is she going to get you in and out of the car? You're a foot taller and outweigh her by seventy pounds."

I already knew the answer to my questions. Joe couldn't even stand, much less walk, and his wife was unable to take him home despite his constant bullying. Joe went quiet, the red slowly draining from his face, his eyes betraying the panic and helplessness he'd tried so hard to hide with his anger.

"Nobody wants to be here, that's only natural. And the staff doesn't want to keep you here. But you need to get stronger so you can go home…safely… successfully. If you go home today and fall, or your wife falls and ends up in the hospital again because she's trying to help you move, you've accomplished nothing except to make your lives more difficult."

I waited a beat and said, "It's your choice."

I had Joe's attention. He could have told me to leave and I would have, allowing him time to digest what I said and keep his pride intact. When someone is angry, it's best to give them space to let the anger die down rather than try to force something to happen or try to dominate the person.

But as it turned out Joe didn't need more space. He was actually ready to have a therapeutic conversation with me regarding how to make the most of a rehab stay in a nursing home.

We had our conversation that day and a few more, and some weeks later Joe completed his rehabilitation and went home with greater strength, able to get out of bed by himself and walk with his walker, no longer dependent on others to assist him with daily tasks.

> We cannot solve our problems with the same thinking
> we used to create them.
> ~ Albert Einstein

As you can see, Joe was trying to solve a new problem – and a big one – with his old ways of thinking and being. He was overbearing as he tried to force the result he wanted and believed was best. It didn't work: Staying with his old ways added to his stress and undermined his recovery. It also upset his disabled wife to the point of tears, and pushed away the staff who felt frustrated and powerless to help him.

Joe's original approach won't work for the rest of us either: When life presents us with something new and challenging, we have to approach it differently or else we'll add to the problem and increase our misery, and add to the misery of those around us.

Here is another example of what happens in skilled nursing rehab. One afternoon I went into a new rehab patient's room, and his roommate yelled out when he saw me, "Listen to her! I didn't and look what happened to me!"

He was right. I had seen Gregg during his previous rehab admission about six months previous and he dismissed everything I suggested, thinking he knew better and nothing applied to him. He was also convinced he wasn't as sick or weak as the doctors and rehab therapists were telling him. So he went home after a few weeks of rehab, still unsteady on his feet but demanding to leave. In his home environment his health quickly went downhill, sending him back to the hospital and to rehab.

Another elderly man in his first rehab stay because of a hip replacement was angry and depressed. After I introduced myself and mentioned how many people I had consulted with during the years, he said, "Good for you!" Then he turned away with a smirk, adding, "I don't need a shrink."

I answered, "I didn't mention how many years' experience in rehab or the number of people I've spoken with to puff myself up, but to let you know I've talked to a lot of people in your exact situation and I've learned what works and what doesn't work. And your attitude doesn't work, and won't get you home any sooner. If you would like me to share that information with you, I'll be glad to."

That got this attention. He listened and did well in rehab. Three weeks later he went home, able to walk throughout the facility and feeling better than he had in a long time.

By the way, I didn't address his "shrink" remark because it would have diverted our focus or set him off into another angry tirade. My primary focus is on what will serve this person in this situation at this moment in time, and enhance their chances of recovery. What I say is tailored to the individual and their circumstances, and on occasion it's best to let some things slide by.

Furthermore, I use the word "information" because it's easier for people to accept. Information is something we often take in, alter to suit our needs and standards, or reject and throw out with the trash. As a result, a little bit of information here and there can go a long way, especially to a mind dulled by illness, pain, medication, emotional distress, and/or dementia.

It's Not What You Expect

So far all my examples have been about some of the men I've met. But women also have difficulty with rehab in a nursing home. The stress of going into a skilled nursing facility for rehabilitation after a serious illness, injury, or surgery hits everyone, male and female, young and old alike. Even those who've had a friend or relative in rehab will be taken aback by their own reactions when it's their turn.

To qualify for rehab, the patient has to have been "admitted" into a hospital for at least three days; it's a Medicare requirement. And those days can't be for just "observation." In addition, the person must be unable to go home due to lack of functional capacity, such as the inability to walk a required amount, or could not get out of bed, and so forth. Sometimes a hospital patient will first be transferred to an inpatient rehab unit for intensive therapy, but they may still need to continue their rehabilitation in a skilled nursing facility in order to have any chance of returning home.

Residents never expect what they encounter either in the hospital or rehab facility. All expect to have uncomplicated hospitalizations and then return home to resume independent living without difficulty. Consequently, patients are surprised when the doctor recommends a transfer to a rehab facility instead of going directly home. This is augmented by the fact they are still not feeling well or even fully aware of what's happening despite repeated explanations by the staff. This is understandable, given their medical status, medications, and possibly anesthesia (more about this later).

As I remind residents and their families, no one is ever ready for this event and no one expects they will become seriously ill and incapacitated, dependent on strangers for assistance with basic bodily functions. And, no one expects they will have to change their lifestyle for the rest of the lives. Residents learn as they go along, since that's the nature of life anyway, but some residents fight their new reality to their detriment, and to the stress of others.

Let's continue with our discussion regarding common rehab challenges and how to deal with them more effectively, whether you're the patient or a family member. Although I'll include some information regarding mental decline and dementia as well as long-term care, the majority of that information will appear in subsequent chapters. In addition, the Appendix includes a Rehab/Skilled Nursing Checklist that I developed over the years, and what I used when my father and husband were in rehab to ensure I didn't overlook important issues.

> Life is what happens while you are busy making other plans.
> ~ John Lennon

Expectations Will Ruin Your Day

Harry retired at age seventy and was now recovering from knee replacement surgery when he was referred to me for depression and not showing enough effort in rehab.

Briefly, if the knee replacement patient is not able to safely walk some fifty feet or so in the hospital or needs quite a bit of help or has complications, they will be transferred to skilled nursing home rehab. This will usually take approximately one to three weeks depending on their age and progress; and up to four weeks for bilateral or double knee replacements. In order to go home, they need to be able to get out of bed or a chair by themselves; go to the bathroom and take care of their needs; manage medications, meals and other basics; and walk several hundred feet. If they can do this, going home will be a success and they will typically continue their recovery with either home health or outpatient physical therapy.

As you would expect, recovery will be quicker the younger and healthier the patient. Old age is a hindrance to successful rehab especially if the patient has other ailments or infections.

Returning to Harry, I found him sitting in a darkened room in the middle of a sunny day, his countenance sullen and gloomy. At first he wasn't in the mood to talk, but he finally opened up.

Harry told me his new knee was hurting after physical therapy, but he was refusing pain medications as well as ice. More importantly, he had expected to go home the day after his surgery. Then he added, "My buddy on my softball team had a knee replacement and told me he was back playing ball in three weeks. Here I am, sitting on my duff, having to ask for help to go to the bathroom. I want to go home and play ball."

First of all, no one, not even Olympic champions in their gold medal prime can return to play softball or any other sport three weeks after a knee replacement. This *does not happen*. Why his buddy said this, or what exactly he said, will remain a mystery;

maybe he was boasting, or trying to paint a rosy picture to encourage Harry. The simple truth – according to rehab specialists – is that this is impossible. One seasoned physical therapist thoughtfully suggested Harry's buddy had probably forgotten what it actually took to rehab his knee. (This is similar to women who forget the pain of a difficult labor and delivery, then choose to get pregnant again after vowing "Never again." It's human nature as well as our survival mechanism, to forget the details of our pain.)

Second, not every knee or other joint replacement, even in the same person, is the same. Not every recovery and rehab is the same, although patterns exist. So comparing oneself to someone else, someone we know nothing about medically, will not serve any helpful purpose. Yet I come across this kind of comparison regularly – and when the mind compares, we're always on the losing side.

Third, Harry's desire to play softball would not come to pass for months at best, if at all. Imagine what it takes to play softball at his advanced age. Also, will his new artificial knee be able to take it and last fifteen to twenty years? Maybe yes, probably not, and I have yet to meet the person who tells me they're looking forward to a repeat joint replacement. We might as well as take good care of the one we have and be realistic about life after joint replacement.

> You got to be careful if you don't know where you're going, because you might not get there.
> ~ Yogi Berra

Harry's main problem and the source of his depression were his **unrealistic expectations** about his surgical recovery. He desperately wanted an easy knee replacement and to return to playing softball quickly. Consequently, he swallowed his buddy's story without a second thought, discounting what his doctor and therapists told him. He expected life, his body, and an artificial knee, to be the way he wanted, but of course, life doesn't play according to our rules. The good news here is Harry ultimately didn't need anti-depressants, because once he corrected his unrealistic expectations and had a new, realistic outlook on rehab, he quickly improved and went home.

Our expectations emerge out of our desires as well as from what we've been taught or what has worked for us in the past (usually in different circumstances). We simply don't question our thoughts about the future or seek out information that confirms, corrects, or refutes our expectations. We assume we're right and never ask the simple question, "Is it true? Are my expectations in line with the reality of my situation?"

If our expectations are not accurate and we don't accept new or contradictory information, disappointment and frustration is guaranteed to follow. As Byron Katie reminds us, "When you argue with reality, you lose, but only 100 percent of the time."

Here's another example of unrealistic expectations and arguing with reality. Stella, a fit and active sixty-seven-year-old woman who just had bilateral knee replacement surgery, told me how she was planning to return to her running program in six weeks so she could run the next 10K race (six miles) in town. I asked her if she had discussed her plan with her orthopedic surgeon, and she answered, "Why should I? What's wrong with running on double knee replacements?"

"If you're planning on running or any other sport that places a lot of force on knee replacements, you ought to discuss it with your surgeon," I answered. "Joint replacements take a long time to completely heal, and you wouldn't want to have a problem and need to have them redone. Talk to your surgeon about your training plans; that race you're telling me about is coming up soon."

Stella looked at me blankly. What I said did not fit in with her expectations and desires – a surefire prescription for Stella to experience more pain and heartache.

More times than I care to remember I'll hear something along the lines of "I read," or, "I heard," or, "My doctor told me I would be healed in three (four, five or six) weeks." Or, "I'll be as good as new when the stitches are taken out (in about ten days)." This is not in keeping with what I've heard from medical professionals, or seen through the years with rehab residents. *As always, the best source of information is your physician and surgeon, not your neighbor or buddy, and certainly not your own unexamined desires.*

The point is to be realistic in your expectations, taking into account your age general health, fitness, activities, as well as what's needed to lead an independent life. Don't be like Harry and blindly listen to a former patient, taking in their story without any thought or reflection. They may be right or partially right, but they could also be wrong.

If you or your loved one is having joint replacement surgery, educate yourself and ask your surgeon for more information so you don't become trapped in the quicksand of false and dangerous expectations.

> Expectation is the root of all heartache.
> ~ Shakespeare

What's Wrong with Perfection?

"See that?" Grace asked with a scowl as she pointed to her bedspread. "They can't do anything right around here. How am I supposed to get better looking at *that* all day?"

"What's exactly is the problem?" I asked, although I already knew since I could see the sloppy corners. But I needed Grace to make it explicit.

"The corners, they're not right!" she huffed, exasperated with me since I obviously couldn't see the problem. "I can't walk and do it myself, and now I have to see it all day."

Grace was eighty-two and slowly recovering from two compressed lumbar factures. She had progressed to the point she could sit in a chair for an hour or two, but walking, bending, and twisting were out of the question.

"Yes, the bedspread could have been folded more carefully. But how important is that on a one to ten scale? How important is it to your recovery?" I asked Grace.

"It's a ten," she quickly answered.

"No, it's not a ten," I said, and waited until we made eye contact. "Let me explain the scale. Ten is life or death, meaning we need to get to an emergency room right now. Eight or nine is pretty close to life or death, like a serious accident or illness, and we need to do something now or the situation will get worse. One is not especially important at all, a passing annoyance like stale coffee. So, the corners not being made right, what number is that?"

Grace went inward, then said, "It's a two."

A little smile came out of hiding, showing me the Grace I had come to know.

"When you get upset about something, ask yourself what number is it from one to ten, and then be upset *up to that number*. No more. We often get upset or angry over something that isn't that important in the grand scheme of life or even rehab, but we never ask ourselves how important is it really?"

Grace nodded when I added, "I've found few things in life are in the eight, nine, or ten zone no matter how they felt at first."

Explaining the Basics so Rehab Isn't Done "Wrong"

"I shouldn't be here. I don't know what happened," said Sally, her skin pale and her hair slightly disheveled. "Is this the hospital?"

Sally, seventy-six-years-young, was a retired, college educated, government manager. She was widowed with one son who lived out of state.

Up until this point, Sally had been living independently in an active retirement community and playing tennis and bridge weekly. She had been in the nursing center a week following the hospitalization for injuries she suffered in a car accident she didn't cause. Sally's right leg had been badly fractured, now held together by rods and screws. She also had a couple of broken ribs and a fractured forearm.

Sally's status was *non-weight bearing*, which meant she was not allowed to stand on her surgically repaired leg. The staff had to repeatedly admonish her not to stand or get out of bed by herself, but she did it anyway, forgetting her leg was fragile until it throbbed. As if that wasn't enough, the staff also said Sally was difficult and short-tempered, repeating the same questions and complaints over and over again. More importantly, Sally was uncooperative with rehab and her medications.

"Good luck," Sally's nurse whispered to me before she hustled out of Sally's room.

"I think they're trying to kill me," Sally said evenly and looked up at me. "Who are you again?"

After introducing myself again, I said, "No, they're not trying to kill you. But you've had a big injury and surgery, and the staff is trying to protect that leg." I pointed to her heavy, full leg brace. "That's why they get after you. You're in a skilled nursing facility for rehabilitation, do you remember what happened to you?"

"A car hit me. I was driving to the mall to get a present for my grandson's graduation. I think he ran a red light...guy who hit me. I don't remember much after that." She shifted uncomfortably in her wheel-chair. "I hate this."

Many "elderly" residents (age sixty-five and up) do not remember what got them to the hospital and rehab, or even where they are presently located. Some do recall what happened prior to their hospitalization, but almost nothing after that. They'll typically say they "woke up in the nursing home" and didn't know what was happening, or whom all the people who came into their room were. They'll also add that no one, including the doctor and family, explained anything to them. Not remembering what happened bothers them, and so I explain that this is a common experience. After all, they've been extremely sick or had surgery, and received pain medications among other drugs and treatments.

In addition, who wants to remember any of this in the first place? When I express this sentiment, they usually agree with me that no one would want to remember a hospital stay and all the misery that entails. Then we move on to what's happening now, and how to get through a rehab stay successfully.

I begin with the basics, going over what happened and where they are, and what the purpose is for being in a skilled nursing home for rehab. Most people do not truly understand what rehab is and are overwhelmed by the related insurance and legal issues. Even though the principal information has already been repeated in one way or another, they can't remember or understand this new world they've been thrown into against their will. The discussion we have allows them to tell their story while we build a therapeutic relationship. Later, I'll explain a few things in language they can hopefully better understand, but first, we get down to basics.

I ask questions and listen – truly listen. This is something that doesn't happen often in the hustle-bustle world of modern healthcare or even in everyday life. I probably already know the resident's pertinent history and primary issues, but everyone needs and deserves to be heard. And if they do feel listened to, trust is fairly easy to build and sets the stage for them to pay attention to my suggestions and work more effectively with the staff.

With Sally, I already knew ten key pieces of information

before we had spoken for five minutes. As always this information applies to more than just Sally and can be used in practical ways, so please don't skip it. Here is **Sally's list**.

1. At seventy-six, Sally was at an age where the body is typically weaker and recovers less quickly, even for someone in relatively good health and fitness level.

2. Sally had a major injury and surgery due to someone else's fault.

3. Sally would probably fall into the "Why me?" dilemma if she hadn't already. (This would prove true, and we dealt with it fairly quickly by correcting her early programming about rewards and punishments.)

Sometimes a resident will come into rehab because they clearly caused the problem that brought them there. As a result, they may wallow in self-blame and criticism. This will hinder a successful rehab as much as "Why me?" thinking and must be addressed. So I tell them we all make mistakes, and some can result in painful, even permanent repercussions. Nevertheless, we must accept responsibility and move forward one step at a time. (What other option is there?)

4. Sally's leg was non-weight bearing, and so her rehab would be longer and slower than most. (No one is ready for that; and no one is ready or expecting a life altering catastrophic event.)

As is often the case, Sally did not fully appreciate what non-weight bearing meant and the safety issues involved. Her rehab would progress slowly until she was cleared for weight bearing status and could begin to put her weight on her leg. This means being able to do required periods of standing, pivoting, more physical therapy, and finally, starting to walk again. Her rehab stay would last many weeks rather than days as most people expect.

5. Sally was probably in considerable pain, which in and of itself can trigger depression. In addition, pain medication she and others take can dull a person's thinking, slow their memory,

and flatten their mood. If someone has never experienced pain or is frightened by it, or is not reacting to pain medication well, this can result in even more challenges. For example, pain medication can also result in constipation – and that makes people uncomfortable and cranky. Residents have been known to go nine days or more without a bowel movement after surgery. Then they will need laxatives, suppositories, and so forth. It is not a pleasant situation, and often quite embarrassing for the residents.

Furthermore, after surgery it is common practice for the patient to receive a course of antibiotics to prevent infection. For the elderly this will usually mean they experience little if any appetite and taste; mild to significant gastrointestinal distress; and a vague sense they are not themselves. They may say they can't "think straight," feel "spacey," and so on. By the way, if an elderly patient develops pneumonia, it usually takes about two months after the end of their antibiotics course for them to "feel like themselves" (this is what actual patients report). As you would expect, their rehab will be long and slow, much to their frustration and worry.

I had noticed too that Sally was shifting in her wheel-chair, which might mean she was developing a sore bottom, or perhaps a painful "bed sore" or a pressure wound in the area of her tailbone. This is not uncommon for the elderly after a hospital stay, since skin gets thinner with age and they may not have been turned (physically) during their hospitalization to relieve pressure on sensitive areas (low back to tailbone and heels). In Sally's case, she might need a better cushioned wheel-chair, a smaller size, or one that did not dip too much in the center. Either way, it's best to ask about this behavior since I've come across residents who are in pain and have not alerted their nurse or therapist.

6. Sally was a smart woman, independent and active, who was used to being in control of her life. This injury had completely

upended her lifestyle and probably would affect the rest of her life. In all likelihood, the aftermath of this injury would also bring an assortment of financial worries, and possibly chronic pain and disability. In addition, Sally probably felt alone, given the fact that she was widowed and her only child lived across the country.

7. Sally did not like being "talked down to," or told what to do. Rather, she was used to being the one who told others what to do, and their job was to do it. This was apparent from both her job history and staff reports.

8. With no known history of dementia, Sally was showing signs of cognitive and memory problems. This was probably scaring her because she could not follow or remember what others told her. Words came and went, and every conversation with staff would seem new and overwhelming. In other words, Sally was still in the dark about what was happening to her and how to best deal with it.

Due to her surgery Sally was given **anesthesia** as well as other drugs. For someone her age, anesthesia can cause mental dullness; impaired attention and concentration; difficulty remembering, reasoning, and making decisions; heightened emotions; internal chilliness; and for a few, even hallucinations (seeing things that others can't see). Some avid readers, for example, will complain they can't read, their concentration wandering so they can't follow the story line or even a caption under a photograph. This will slowly improve over the first few weeks, but the impairment can last up to six to eight weeks. And, for a small percentage of elderly residents, it can be permanent.

In addition, hospitalized elderly patients over age sixty-five are more prone to develop **delirium** which can co-exist with dementia and/or is often misdiagnosed as dementia or Alzheimer's (which develop gradually). Delirium comes on quickly and probably has multiple causes, including the aftermath of surgery. It is *a sudden and significant impairment in mental abilities* *and can include an inability to focus, poor memory and speech, confusion, agitation and even combativeness, hallucinations, delusions, and extreme emotions.* The condition can fluctuate, with periods of withdrawal with little or no activity and responsiveness. If you have concerns about delirium and your loved one is in a hospital or nursing home, please discuss it with their nurse or physician. If you can, provide a concise history of the patient's functioning prior to admission since this will aid diagnosing. As a family member, be patient since delirium can take some time to resolve.

9. In all likelihood Sally's sleep was disturbed due to pain, the inability to move her braced leg into a comfortable position, and/or having to sleep in a new position in a new bed in a new room with people coming and going. If she was receiving sleep medication, that could result in side effects such as drowsiness, headaches, and a dulled mind. In addition, for some people pain medication can disrupt sleep or impede falling asleep, cause itching or disturbing dreams, which wake them up.

As if that isn't enough, nursing homes run on a 24/7 clock so lights will be turned on and staff will speak at normal volume – not whispers – even in the middle of the night. Sally will be woken up for medications; to be routinely examined and checked on; have diapers, clothing and bedding to be changed if needed; or, to get blood drawn (which happens in the wee hours of the morning), and so on. And if Sally is lucky enough to bypass all of this, her roommate or other nearby residents won't, and their care could wake her up. Moreover, if residents do not get enough sleep they will often be in low spirits, irritable, prickly, and certainly in no mood to go to therapy or cooperate with staff.

10. Sally, like any other new rehab resident, was extremely stressed, and as a result, her fundamental emotional patterns would show. This meant anxiety, heightened frustration, short-temperedness, suspiciousness, and distrust of what she could not understand. This resulted in refusals of therapy and medication

as well as strained relationships with staff and other residents.

In short, Sally was not at her best and well on her way to doing rehab "wrong." *Then again, who is their best under the circumstances?* I write the latter not to excuse "bad" or uncooperative behavior, but rather to open our minds and hearts to a greater understanding of what someone is going through, and from there figure out how to best address it and support them.

> Compassion is love with understanding,
> where there is no judgment.
> ~ Sai Maa

Understanding the Influence of Past Issues: Compassionate Listening

Here's how a past experience and a fear-based program can undermine rehab and look like a lack of cooperation when it is not.

Years ago an elderly man came into rehab following a stroke. John was a small, thin fellow who rarely spoke, hardly ate, and stayed in his room, sitting by the window. He often refused therapy or if he did go, did very little. He was described by staff as "extremely nervous" and as someone who "didn't seem to understand what was happening." It seemed no one could communicate with him enough to find out what the problem was.

I found an anxious, shy man who didn't say much and seemed confused and unable to concentrate. Although his medical condition had stabilized and he didn't have any known infections, I wondered whether his stroke was bigger and his mind was more scrambled than what the doctors thought, perhaps made worse by undiagnosed dementia or an undiscovered medical problem. My first goal was to be gentle and soft-spoken, and try to make a connection with John so I could figure out what was making him so scared and withdrawn. A stoke is scary, and finding yourself stuck in a rehab center can be overwhelming and confusing, but this had a different flavor and was more pronounced.

As we spoke about John's past, he made a passing comment that he was drafted into the Army at age eighteen and sent into combat in Europe during World War II. A short time later, he was captured and spent a year in a German POW (prisoner of war) camp. While John said this, he became visibility more anxious, and I wondered if his confinement in the rehab center, surrounded by people he could not understand and who dictated his every move, was triggering his POW trauma.

Aware I had to calm down his fear and do it that day so his rehab participation would improve, I decided to use John's POW experience as a template. I explained to him where he was, what was he doing there, who the people were who came and went from his room. Most of the staff spoke in accented English he couldn't understand and repeatedly told him what to do, prompting John to ask me whether the staff was out to "hurt him." Thankfully, by that point something had "clicked" between us, and John trusted me and my explanation that they were medical personnel there to ensure his safety and work with him on his recovery. From that point on, John's fear and anxiety decreased, and he began to do his rehab well.

Every week I'd go over the same basic information with John to quell his fears and encourage him. A few weeks later I finally had the chance to speak with his wife, who confirmed John had been diagnosed with "Battle Fatigue" (now known as PTSD or Post-Traumatic Stress Syndrome) and had experienced symptoms all his adult life. Ultimately John went home, still a shy man, but much stronger and calmer, and almost fully recovered from his stroke.

This is an example as well as a lesson that we never know all the factors influencing a human being or how they are behaving as a patient. As a result, we must learn to listen carefully and compassionately, open to the idea that old programming and traumas can be affecting their present behavior and recovery.

In summary, if your mother, father, spouse or partner, brother, sister, or other loved one is going through a health crisis that lands them in a skilled nursing facility, use **Sally's list** as a resource to come up with one that is individual to them. Then use your list to problem solve and support them. Modify the list as time goes on, since situations, issues, and conditions change.

Also, use the list daily to prepare yourself to visit your infirmed loved one. This will help you drop your expectations that they will be their usual self or how you think a (perfect) rehab patient should be.

In the next chapter, we'll go into greater depth regarding what happens in rehab, the issues residents and families face, and ways to handle this unique situation more effectively. If you are about to undergo elective surgery, such as a knee or hip replacement, use the information in these chapters as well as the Rehab/Skilled Nursing Checklist to prepare yourself.

> When you get into a tight place and everything goes against you, till it seems as though you could not hang on a minute longer, never give up… for that is just the place and time that the tide will turn.
> ~ Harriet Beecher Stowe

Time-Tested Tips

- If you have a "Joe" on your hands who is belligerent and demanding to go home, get professional help and please don't wait. Precious rehab time is slipping away because Medicare and/or other insurance cover a limited number of rehab days.

- Got a new problem? Be like Einstein and change your thinking. Change how you approach the problem if your current tactic is not working.

- Remind yourself that rehab is stressful, multi-faceted, and never as easy as it looks or others say. Listen to the resident and remember they are probably in pain as well as scared or worried.

- Educate yourself regarding rehab. Consider new information. There is a wealth of information available on the internet or your nearest library computer. It's up to you whether you make it harder than it needs to be or easier on yourself and your family.

- Are your expectations helping or hurting you? What are your expectations?

- Make a list. It will enlighten you in ways you cannot imagine or predict.

- Rate an upset or problem from one to ten. Then be upset up to that number *and no more.*

- As you'll see in the next chapter, rehab is not a vacation or a time to simply rest and recuperate as some think. A resident's energy is needed for rehab therapies as well as for the body to recuperate. So, there will be little time or energy for pleasure reading, hobbies, visitors, etc.

- Breathe deeply and slowly at least three times in a row. Do it every day, and do it often during stressful times to discover and anchor your peace.

When life doesn't make sense, we can still have peace.
~ Rick Warren

Chapter 3
Getting Rehab Right

Now that we are more aware of expectations and old patterns that interfere with our recovery or our support of a loved one's recovery, let's figure out how to help ourselves and others during rehab. Below are a series of questions I typically use to learn how a resident is faring in rehab, followed by the most important recommendations to help them succeed. The recommendations notwithstanding, getting rehab right is as much about having the right attitude and understanding as it is about doing physical exercises, taking medication, and so on.

<blockquote>
All beginnings are difficult.
~ Talmud
</blockquote>

Question #1: "What happened? What brought you into rehab?"

It's important the resident gets to tell their story; so I ask them what happened. The tale of what went "wrong," or what needed fixing, is something they'll usually repeat again and again. That's fine as long as they don't get stuck in "broken record" storytelling that does not lead to a resolution. If this occurs, at some point I tell them we need to move on and deal with what's happening right now, so they can complete rehab and go home.

That's the goal: recover from the illness or surgery; get stronger and improve everyday living skills; and return home safely. Neither the nursing home nor the staff wants new rehab residents to remain in the nursing home for the rest of their lives. If that's what happens because there is no other option because of a chronic medical condition and its disability, so be it, but that is not the goal of rehab. It may seem unnecessary to emphasize the goal of a rehab stay, but many residents worry they're going to remain in the nursing home forever or that the nursing home only wants to keep them for the money.

Question #2: "How do you feel physically? Are you hurting? If yes, where? When does it hurt, and when did it start?"

Let nursing know if your resident complains of pain because it's possible they have not told anyone they're in pain, or informed them how much or how often. They may need a change in their medication or its scheduling, ice to quell inflammation, or a consult with a specialist or surgeon. Or, the resident may need further education as to what to expect, including pain and discomfort, with their joint replacement or other surgery. Accurate information alone is sometimes enough to allay their fears and decrease their pain level.

Sometimes residents say they don't want to request pain medications because they don't want "to bother" the nurses or become addicted. I answer that the staff is there to help them, that's what they're being paid to do. In addition, it's the staff's job to help regardless of their demeanor or attitude, or whether they're acting rushed or attentive and considerate.

It's also important that a patient not take staff reactions, facial expressions or even their words personally, because if they do, they'll suffer even more. In psychology this is called *personalization* whereby we take others' negative behaviors as solely pertaining to us and signifying something significant and negative about our self-worth. As a result, it is important to emphasize that the reactions of others are about themselves, not the resident.

When all is said and done, staff behavior and reactions will come and go. They are just a result of human nature showing itself. This is not to say that abuse or disrespect of any resident should be tolerated – not at all. But when a resident speaks about "not bothering staff," they are showing their old programming about being the "good" girl or boy. This may involve beliefs that they shouldn't voice their needs or put anyone out; shouldn't hurt someone's feelings; and/or, they should be strong and self-reliant. I remind rehab residents they're in the nursing home to get rehabilitated, and that needs to be *their number one priority*. Pleasing others has to remain outside of the rehab equation. Even the most ardent people-pleasers must learn this fact to successfully recover.

Residents recovering from surgery and other painful conditions need a little help, or they will not be able to successfully complete rehab if they remain stressed and overwhelmed by pain. If they try to "tough it out" at their age – which some try to do since that's been a pattern in their life – it's counterproductive, as well as physically and emotionally taxing. Also keep in mind the doctors and pharmacy consultants oversee a resident's pain medications to ensure residents are not over-medicated and do not get addicted. As a result, becoming addicted to pain medications while in rehab is basically a non-issue.

In addition, for pain medications to work effectively, it's important to remain "ahead of the pain." That is, *patients should not wait until pain is at an excruciating level because that will hinder the medication's effectiveness*. Although there are several effective pain management techniques (see Resources section in the Appendix), elderly rehab residents usually cannot follow them enough to do them. Even younger residents will shy away from using these techniques. Consequently, pain medications play a necessary role in a rehab center. Of course, it's important to monitor the resident for the side effects of pain medication, especially the elderly. If you have any concerns, please speak to their nurse or physician.

Lastly, the 4 - 4 Breathing technique can also be used as a simple pain management method assuming it is used regularly and correctly. It works as a pain management technique because if the mind-body becomes more relaxed, pain generally begins to subside, alleviating the suffering.

Question #3: "How are you sleeping?"

The elderly recovering resident may not need eight hours a night, but they do need enough undisturbed sleep so they can rest and recover. The issue is whether they are getting a restful night's sleep, whatever that means for them individually. Some residents, however, will sleep more during their recovery, and that's generally not a problem unless it's interfering with their rehab therapies or reflects an unresolved medical issue.

If the resident is taking sleep medications, monitor for side effects that may be hampering their rehab such as lowered energy and mood, as well as mental or cognitive decline.

Question #4: "How's your appetite? How much are you eating?"

If the elderly rehab resident eats about half of what is on their meal tray without losing weight, they're probably doing fine because they will usually be served larger portions than they are used to. Moreover, when they're sick a full plate may seem overwhelming and unappetizing. As a result, it is usually not necessary that they "clean their plates."

Residents often complain about nursing home food: It's either "unseasoned" or "too seasoned," has "too much salt or gravy," or has "too much chicken." Or, the meat is "too tough," the portions "too big," "vegetables are overcooked," and so on. Keep in mind that it's institutional food and not home cooking tailored specifically for the preferences of those living at home. Nevertheless, the food seems to serve the majority of residents well enough to aid their recovery.

Some residents may be on a special diet. Or they may need to receive chopped or pureed food, or need liquids thickened to aid swallowing. No one likes this and so the residents often complain, but it may be necessary given their health condition. If there are any food or nutrition concerns you or the resident has, please discuss with the dietician, nurse, or physician.

In addition, if their caloric intake is being supplemented with protein shakes, it's best that these are not drunk close to meal times. Protein shakes are filling, and residents will push away their meals as a result.

Rehab residents and families sometimes complain there are few salads and fresh fruits served. The reason for this is straightforward: Elderly residents do not eat these items in sufficient quantities to justify the cost. These (and much of the food served) end up being thrown away. But, if the resident wants and will eat fruit and salads, or is vegetarian, contact the dietician to discuss options.

Doctors say we lose about half of our taste buds by the age of fifty, and antibiotics and other medications can interfere with appetite and taste. Basically, food will taste like cardboard, and be about as appealing as a bowl of sawdust. To counteract the resident's reduced appetite and complaints, some family members and friends bring sugary snacks and junk food to a rehab resident. Sometimes visitors bring in so many snacks and sweets they are piled high on the bedside tables, and if they can't be completely closed these will attract ants or other critters. More importantly, residents need nutritious food, especially proteins, for their recovery.

An example of non-nutritious food is the resident who had a gallon can of bubble gum brought in by her husband which triggered an eating binge of sweets. By law, the nursing home was powerless to restrict her gum and other sweets due to resident rights. This resident gained twenty pounds over the course of her stay which did not help her new knee and recovery from an infection.

So, if family or friends want to bring food, check first with the nurse or dietician to make sure it won't go against any dietary restrictions. Then bring something the resident likes – in small portions. Make sure it also smells good in order to stimulate the senses and appetite. Or, consider bringing low sugar protein bars or other healthy snacks. If they don't want it, let it be. Don't push, nag, or coax because it'll probably be heard as a criticism and that they're not pleasing you, resulting in unnecessary conflict and even reduced cooperation with staff and rehab.

Question #5: "How much water are you drinking?" (*Check first to see if they're on fluid restriction.)

As we age we drink less and less water to the point some elderly residents only drink a few ounces a day, and only when they're taking medication. However, the human body and our cells need water, and water helps flush toxins from the body. Therefore, during rehab it's best to drink several glasses of water per day if possible. However, if the doctor has placed a water or fluid restriction for medical reasons, then stick to that amount in order to help the body recover.

Some rehab residents will avoid drinking water because they do not want to ask for help to go to the bathroom, or are worried if they do have to go, they will have to wait too long for help to arrive and will urinate on themselves beforehand. Others will try to go to the bathroom by themselves, either forgetting they can't or not wanting to wait for help. When this happens, I suggest they look at this situation from a practical, safety point of view and not as a dignity or self-esteem issue. Yes, they can get up and try to walk ten feet to the bathroom, like they've done all their lives. But if they stumble – and it's easy to stumble if the body is weak or a little slow from illness and/or the effects of medication – they can easily fall and break a hip, bone, or vertebrae.

In view of that, I ask what they would rather experience, a broken hip or wetting themselves and the bed? Of course nobody likes to wet themselves; it's an insult to our adult pride. And no one, staff included, likes having to change the bed and clothing, especially in the middle of the night. But changing the resident and their bed takes about twenty minutes, while a broken hip will mean surgery, hospitalization, and a painful rehab on top of whatever rehab they now have. The majority of residents see the practical wisdom in this approach and stop trying to go to the bathroom by themselves.

Sometimes family or a new resident complain about the resident having to wear diapers, saying this is a "dignity issue" (e.g., no adult should wear diapers). They want the aides to respond quickly every time the resident needs to go to the bathroom, but this is impossible, given the number of residents per aide. There are three options in this scenario, none of which the resident or their family finds appealing. First, the family hires (expensive) private duty aides 24/7 so there will always be someone available to take their loved one the bathroom. Few residents or their family can afford this option. Second, family takes the resident home so they can provide a higher standard of care. However, this is often not physically, emotionally, or economically possible. Third, accept that some residents, whether in rehab or long-term care, need to wear diapers. This will entail changing one's definition of what is a dignity issue and what is a medical necessity.

I sometimes suggest residents look at wearing diapers or pull-ups, having to use a bedpan, or depending on strangers to help them to the bathroom from the point of view of a small child. That is, urination and bowel movements are just nature at work, an essential part of having a human body and something we all need to do regularly. If you spend time with toddlers, you'll notice they'll continue playing without a thought about dignity when their diapers are wet or poop is falling out. This is because they haven't learned this is unacceptable and undignified. For adults, when we get sick and disabled or when women give birth, modesty, privacy, and dignity related to bodily functions flies out the window. Then we have no choice but to change our thinking and accept the reality of how a human body and medical care interact.

Some older female residents, however, balk at having a male aide take them to the bathroom, help them change or shower. This was a totally unacceptable concept in their early life and they cannot get used to the idea in their later years. Also, at times a resident does not get along with their aide. These situations can be remedied by requesting a change to a female aide. Fortunately, most facilities can accommodate this request readily.

Another common issue related to water intake is **Urinary Tract Infection** (UTI). This infection can develop quickly and without the usual symptoms a younger adult notices. In the elderly and infirmed, the effects can be pronounced, including significant mental decline and confusion from one day to the next. The resident may appear as if they have mid-to-late stage dementia when in fact they do not. A UTI usually resolves quickly once a known infection is addressed with antibiotics. However, it is important to bear in mind there are other reasons for a mental decline, even a sudden deterioration. Nevertheless, for elderly residents, it's usually recommended they drink more water and fluids in general, even additional cranberry juice or capsules if needed and tolerated for a UTI. As always consult with their physician, nurse practitioner, or physician assistant. Please keep in mind this brief overview is for educational purposes only and does not take the place of medical evaluation and treatment.

Question #6: "Do you drink alcohol? Do you take any drugs not prescribed by your doctor? Do you smoke?"

Over the counter (OTC) medications, smoking, **alcohol and recreational/street drugs** can play a significant role in a resident's rehab and recovery. Keep in mind that OTCs and supplements are typically not allowed in a nursing facility unless they are prescribed and/or approved by a physician. Any questions or concerns should be addressed to the nurse and attending physician.

Alcohol presents unique issues with elderly rehab patients. Some residents were drinking alcohol, sometimes heavily, prior to their admission to the hospital. As a result, they come into the nursing home having completed the first phase of detox while in the hospital, but are still detoxing at admission to rehab. Because of their chronic alcohol use, they may exhibit mental and psychological impairments for a significant period of time on top of their medical problems.

Here's an example: One eighty-year-old with "mild cognitive

impairment" was not improving as expected and eating very little. At times he refused his rehab therapies or put out little effort, jeopardizing his recovery. One day an aide took his water cup to refill it; as it turned out his cup was filled with vodka and orange juice. This was the "lunch" the resident had been having in rehab – every day. In addition, the staff discovered vodka in his closet in a disguised bottle. Apparently this gentleman and his elderly demented wife drank approximately 8 ounces of vodka for lunch every day, and then more alcohol in cocktails later in the day. When staff asked his middle-aged daughter how he got the vodka, she answered, "Daddy asked me to bring him some." Showing *her* early programming, she brought her father the vodka he wanted without a second thought. This resident did much better in rehab once his alcohol was removed, although he complained loudly the nursing home didn't have the right to take away his vodka.

One wealthy seventy-five-year-old woman came into rehab following a fall, as well as declining health and weight loss. The hospital noted alcohol addiction, which she vehemently denied, saying, "We (my husband and I) drank socially all our lives. Cocktails every evening. I'm not a drunk on the street who can't function." Yet, her cognition, memory, poor motivation and slow progress in rehab, as well as what little social history the facility unearthed, contradicted her. Every day she proclaimed she "hated" the nursing home and wanted to go home, adding that she "…couldn't wait for her five o'clock cocktail."

As women alcoholics age, their bodies will show the detrimental effects of alcoholism earlier than men. Although the facility can address detox symptoms, anxiety and depression, the addiction itself is not a focus of treatment in rehab since a skilled nursing home is not geared for this type of treatment, and the resident is still medically sick and mentally impaired. If the resident can do their rehab and progress, they will regain some measure of health and strength. Then upon discharge, they will still need to address their need for treatment for their addiction.

Those residents who deny their problem and return to their old drinking habits once they are discharged, will likely experience more medical problems, including falls, followed by repeat hospitalizations and rehab admissions. The facility can make recommendations and referrals, but it's up to the resident, hopefully with the help of family and addiction specialists, to follow through.

Here's another example of how alcoholism can show up during rehab. A seventy-year-old man with Parkinson's and the beginning of dementia was making slow but steady progress in his rehab. While discussing his upcoming discharge, his wife of almost fifty years mentioned she was worried he would resume drinking, since he was already talking about drinking once he got home. However, this was the first time anyone in the facility had heard of his alcoholism! This fact was not in his available medical history, and a resident *never* reports alcoholism or drug addiction unless they are active in AA or a similar program. In addition, this wife said she could never say "No" to him or refuse to get his booze because he would become angry and verbally abusive. Then she added that he "…also had a stash of guns and ammunition in the house."

I recommended she immediately get rid of the guns since alcoholism, coupled with dementia and its impaired judgment and impulse control, as well as his long-standing short-fuse anger, could easily lead to reckless gunfire. She removed the guns, and in conjunction with the discharge planner, the resident was later transferred to a memory care ALF.

Although this scenario is a bit extreme, it is common for elderly wives (and mothers) to say that they "have to" comply with their infirmed husband's (or adult son or daughter, mostly son's) requests and demands for alcohol and/or money they know will be used to buy alcohol and street drugs. Because of their upbringing and early programming, these women cannot conceive of ever refusing these demands even though the resident cannot drive or otherwise get their alcohol or drugs on their own, and the infirmed loved one can only harm them with their words. In their minds (and early programming), these women think their job as wives and mothers is to please and take care of family, especially their husband or father, and helping does not include setting hard limits. ***Know that when dementia is thrown into the mix, addictions, guns, and impulsive choices can lead to deadly consequences.***

Recreational or street drugs will also result in earlier-than-expected health problems, as well as interfere with medications, treatments, and rehab. For example, I know about some residents who were actively using street drugs, whether so called "mild" or "recreational" drugs or more hard core drugs, prior to their hospitalization and rehab admission. A few of these have met friends outside the facility in order to get these drugs or return from an outing "high" or "under the influence." Skilled nursing homes are *not* detox or alcohol and drug treatment facilities, and are not equipped to handle an active addict. In addition, these residents can be irritable, demanding, and uncooperative, as well as mentally impaired in one way or another for a significant period of time due to their long-standing addiction.

In the coming decades, the Baby Boomers – the first generation to grow up with readily available recreational/street drugs – will arrive in rehab in greater numbers. Consequently, drug addiction and its aftermath will become an enormous problem for skilled nursing facilities. The typical nursing home is geared to handle elderly residents suffering medical issues, not younger, active poly-drug addicts and alcoholics with serious medical conditions, poor lifestyle choices, negative attitudes, and few, if any, support systems. In all probability, society will have to provide specialized facilities or units with specially trained staff for this population.

Restrictions also apply to smoking which most facilities no longer allow on their campuses, and this may include a ban on e-cigarettes and the like. Some smokers give up their habits once confronted with a chronic, debilitating illness, while others return to smoking once they are discharged. In some cases, when a rehab resident who smokes begins to feel better, they may request and even demand they be allowed to smoke. Residents have even been caught smoking in their bathrooms. If your loved one is a smoker and has no desire to quit, it's probably best they go to a rehab facility that allows smoking or the use of e-cigarettes to avoid ongoing conflict.

It must be remembered that skilled nursing homes are medical facilities geared toward rehabilitation and must follow strict standards that sometimes go against personal desires and addictions. If your loved one drinks, smokes, uses drugs or has a history of addiction, especially an active one, please alert the social worker, nursing staff, or attending physician immediately. This is necessary because it is very possible the facility has no record of their addictive history since the only information a facility gets comes from the hospital and it is always limited.

In addition, if a new resident has been using alcohol, drugs, or cigarettes recently and/or long-term, they will undergo a detoxing process as their body and brain clears these toxic substances. They will probably exhibit impaired mental abilities, poor judgment, and weak impulse control as well as emotional ups and downs (which may improve as their brain clears). However, the more complete detox from drugs and alcohol can take many months, and skilled nursing rehab rarely lasts that long.

Question #7: "Do you understand what rehab is? Tell me what you know."

Most residents, unless they've been in rehab before, have no idea what rehab is or what it involves. In addition, they're probably not thinking or remembering clearly, so what they heard yesterday or an hour ago could be long gone. If you want to know if a resident with any kind of cognitive impairment understands you, do not go by their nonverbal language such as head nods, smiles, or even eye contact. Rather, ask them to repeat what they've heard, if they are still able to talk. This can show us how much or how little they actually understood and retained.

> We must be willing to let go of the life we planned, so
> as to have the life that is waiting for us.
> ~ E.M. Forster

Question #8: "How do you feel emotionally? What's your biggest worry this week?"

The focus of skilled nursing rehab is to assist the resident in recovering their health and functional, independent living abilities. As discussed previously, the new resident is likely experiencing adjustment issues due to multiple stressors, and they may well exhibit long-standing negative habits and traits. Once in a while a family will request psychological services because they think their parent or loved one needs a personality makeover. This may well be true, but if the resident has not requested psychotherapy for this purpose and cannot meaningfully participate due to age, illness, or dementia – it's not going to work.

Short-term rehab cannot solve all the resident's health or life issues, or change their personality. Our main focus is solely on getting them through their rehab as best as humanly possible and returning them home.

As part of their adjustment, many rehab residents experience an early bout of **depression**. This is understandable, given the traumatic events that happened to them in a short period of time, including the stress of illness or surgery, pain, anesthesia effects, impaired mobility, and insurance and financial worries. These problems are multi-faceted and not easily resolved, and some could well last the rest of their life. However, if the residents can move through this "situational depression" fairly quickly and it does not significantly interfere with their rehab progress, there is no pressing need for anti-depressants.

But there are times the resident's mood will not improve, and they may cry easily, worry incessantly, lack rehab motivation, or refuse to do for themselves. As a result, their rehab and recovery suffers. Clinical research from the past several decades indicates depression will adversely affect health and immune functioning, as well as lead to or exacerbate chronic pain. Furthermore, there are times when psychological interventions alone cannot overcome the combined effect of multiple stressors and serious physical conditions. When this happens, anti-depressant medication needs to be considered and a referral to a psychiatrist or the attending physician is made. Of course, the resident's other medications as well as their medical condition will need to be taken into account before any anti-depressant is prescribed.

Some families refuse to consider anti-depressants because they fear side effects or they do not like the idea of an anti-depressant, often saying they don't want their loved one to be "dopey" or "out of it." Some older residents also refuse, seeing the use of an anti-depressant as reflecting a character defect or weakness. Others think they can take them, but only when they feel "down in the dumps" and "need it." But anti-depressants do not work this way and need to be taken consistently over a period of time. If the depression is not resolving or is threatening the resident's rehab, yet they or their family have concerns about its safety, they need to discuss this further with their physician, physician assistant, or nurse practitioner. If the resident and/or their family decides against an anti-depressant, this means it'll be up to the elderly, infirmed resident to overcome their depression, and this may be difficult even with the best non-medication psychological interventions.

Sometimes a resident is admitted into rehab and their mood and depression worsens by the day. They become increasingly listless and may cry for no apparent reason they or the staff can identify. Then we find out the resident has been on anti-depressant medication for some time, even years, and it was discontinued in the hospital. In these cases, their body and mind are reacting to the sudden withdrawal of the anti-depressant, and they need their medication. This is one of the many reasons *to keep a current list of medications the resident was taking **before** they got sick, as well as keep track of changes to their medications **in the hospital***. This will help the nursing home staff help your loved one. Remember, the information a nursing home receives from the hospital will be the last medication list and the discharge summary and/or H & P (History & Physical), and not a detailed pre-hospital medical or medication history.

One scenario that still occurs (although much less often than in previous years) is the elderly resident who's placed on strong sedating medications in the hospital to control extreme agitation, aggression, pulling out intravenous lines, and the like. Once in the skilled nursing home, these medications must be closely monitored and decreased as soon as possible to avoid the continuing use of "anti-psychotics" long after residents need them. In my early years in nursing homes I would see this fairly often: The resident, both in rehab and later in long-term care, would still be receiving anti-psychotic medication because of an old hospital diagnosis and prescription, and no current psychiatrist available to titrate these drugs down.

Question #9: "Do you wish you were dead? Are you feeling suicidal?"

If your body is hurting enough for long enough and you can't do for yourself, it is not uncommon for a resident to feel like they want to die and check out of their body and the situation. This is true regardless of the resident's age. The younger residents will fear a long life of infirmity and pain, and want out. The older person will say they've lived a long life and given the circumstances, they'd rather die. If their health situation improves though, this feeling passes, reflecting that it was a *by-product of how they felt **physically**, as well as what they expect and what they think about the situation.*

This was true for Sally (who we met in Chapter 2) following a serious car accident. Shortly after her admission, Sally began wishing she would die quickly and painlessly, but she had no plan or means to harm herself. After all, how much could Sally actually do with her leg in a heavy brace? What means were at her disposal?

This is *passive suicidal ideation*, and what we see most commonly in nursing and rehab facilities. Like Sally, most residents get through this with targeted interventions and proceed onward with rehab. Rarely will a resident actually have any kind of a plan, much less the means and opportunity to actually attempt to harm themselves. Nevertheless, this wish to die and the underlying depression fueling it must be addressed.

Once in a while a resident will express a wish to die or to kill themselves, later saying it was said "in jest" or "out of frustration and they didn't mean it." They are surprised the nursing staff took it seriously and a psychologist or psychiatrist was called in. However, *in a healthcare facility, every suicidal comment, no matter how passive or lacking in intent, opportunity or means, will be taken seriously.*

One sixty-eight-year-old resident added that although her statement of "...wanting to slit her throat" was made in jest, it arose from the fact she'd been dwelling on all the opportunities to do certain activities that were now gone from her life forever. When, as part of our dialog, I suggested she focus not on what she had lost (only one recent activity in which she was an ancillary participant), but on her rehab so she could do more in the future, she shook her head and repeated her belief, "...all was lost in her life." This pointed not to active suicidal thinking since she had no real plan or intention, but to a long-standing depression where life was always "the glass half empty" and she could not imagine a "glass half full."

> You are living or dying every moment with your
> choices. You are constantly choosing dying which is
> fear, or living which is love.
> ~ Sai Maa

Some rehab residents will ruminate about wanting to die to end their suffering, even asking me if the doctor will "help" them. This is not possible. Furthermore, it is not their time to die because they do not have a terminal condition that is (medically) expected to cause death soon. They are in the nursing home for *rehab* and so the goal is to get them *better* so they can go home. Even for the small number of rehab residents who have a terminal condition, their rehab goals remain essentially the same as those who are not terminal. This is so because once they get stronger and are discharged, they will be scheduled for chemotherapy or other treatments to help them in their fight.

A small number of elderly residents will be adamant they do not want the medical interventions they're receiving and wish to die. I sometimes ask them if their true desire is to die a quick death, then why did they consent to surgeries and other intensive treatments? Some tell me they didn't consent at all; that the doctors did it "on their own." I remind them that doctors and hospitals need consent for all treatment, especially surgery, so they (the resident), their legal representative or next of kin, must have agreed and done so in writing.

In addition, if they nevertheless want to stop treatments, medications, dialysis, and/or surgery, they need to discuss this with their families as well as their doctor to make their wishes known and set forth in writing. After all, skilled nursing facilities and rehab are not prisons established to torment patients for profit (despite how some residents view them). Yet, in my over twenty years of working in nursing homes, only a handful of residents have taken steps to curtail medical interventions that are keeping them alive. Most simply want to feel better and whatever problems they're facing resolved as if by magic, rather than confront serious life-or-death medical decisions head-on. (See Chapter 10 for more information regarding end-of-life issues and decision-making.)

Lastly, if an alert resident is persistent in their belief that now is their time to die and they're unmotivated to do rehab, I'll sometimes say, "You're obviously not dying today, this moment. Right?"

They nod agreement to that basic fact, puzzled by what I've said.

"So, it's not your time to die," I'll add, and they'll nod their heads.

"How do I know it's not your time to die?" I ask them.

After a moment or two they'll say, "Because I'm not dead."

"That's right. Here you are with us for rehab, already better medically because you've been discharged from the hospital and sent here. The real issue right now is whether or not you're going to do your rehab." And with that we can move on to how to do rehab right.

> Life just happens. It's what you're believing about life
> that makes you suffer.
> ~ Byron Katie

Time-Tested Tips

- If you're going into rehab because of elective surgery or you find yourself managing the care of a loved one, use the Rehab/Skilled Nursing checklist in the Appendix to guide you. Modify the checklist as necessary since every situation is different, and issues will change over time.

- Be aware of your expectations and correct them as needed. What is reality telling you as opposed to what you are thinking or saying about reality?

- If a resident is having psychological or adjustment issues, or is not participating enough in their rehab, request a mental health consult. Sometimes family wait too long and will even refuse psychological services until rehab is about to be terminated due to lack of participation. Medicare and other third party payers will only pay for so much rehab, so address these issues in a timely fashion, preferably early on since it is easier to right a ship that is beginning to stray off course than turn the ship around. If a resident is referred early enough, many times I'll only need to see a resident 1-3 times in order to address an escalating poor attitude, erroneous expectations, poor adjustment, or low rehab participation.

- Keep in mind that it is not your job to be the resident's psychologist. Don't ask all the questions covered in this chapter or try to assess their mental health. These were included for educational purposes to highlight common issues, not as a psychotherapy "to do list."

- If your resident is voicing a wish to die, here are a few key points to further guide your understanding and response. Please note that I am <u>not</u> suggesting family ask or assess whether their loved one is suicidal. Nonetheless, family do sometimes ask and discuss this issue with their loved one prior to alerting staff, so keep this information in mind.

  If your loved one has voiced a wish to die, do not ask them, "Do you want to die?" This phrasing is confrontational and will likely result in "No" because it's too direct and momentarily takes the resident out of their emotions and into more conscious thinking. By answering "No," the resident is trying to avoid upsetting the family member/questioner, deflect argument and criticism, and/or not go against religious training. It's very possible the resident is experiencing medical problems, significant pain, or deepening depression and fear that needs to be addressed. Yet this question and their "No" will stop any further investigation or needed intervention. If your loved one voices a wish to die or harm themselves in any way, please alert their nurse, social worker, or physician as soon as possible and let them assess the situation.

  In almost all cases it has been my experience that the elderly rehab resident *wishes* to die, but does not want to do anything actively to bring about their death. This is a passive wish to be finished with pain and suffering, preferably dying in their sleep, rather than active decision-making about ending their life or medical treatments. However, as stated previously, every suicidal comment, no matter how passive or lacking in intent, opportunity or means, or whether said in jest and out of frustration, will and should be taken seriously.

- **4 - 4 Breathing:** Breathe deeply and slowly at least three times in a row. Do it every day, and do it often during stressful times to discover and anchor your peace.

> All the world is full of suffering.
> It is also full of overcoming.
> ~ Helen Keller

Chapter 4
The Rehab Roller-coaster

Rehab is a puzzle for the resident, and often for their family as well. There are expectations from every quarter, and plenty of unanswered questions and worries. Every day rehab residents are expected to do a variety of things with virtually no allowance made for the fact they are sick, weak, and helpless. This is an even more pressing issue as the authorized number of days in rehab is decreasing, and residents must improve more quickly.

Residents are understandably frustrated and self-critical when they cannot easily perform tasks and exercises they are expected to do. Some react with outright anger and bossiness, while others become fretful, needy, or demanding. Others feel "bad" or upset, even embarrassed and ashamed they cannot live up to expectations and have to depend on others for everyday activities such as going to the bathroom.

This ongoing experience stimulates negative self-talk and self-criticism that robs residents of any "get up and go." They'll begin to feel dejected and hopeless, unable to get motivated and focus on their rehab. Often, they'll voice a sense of inner shame, as well as exhibit "What's the use?" thinking.

"What's the use of working hard in rehab (when it's not going to get me better or get me home)?"

"Why bother (when I've lost my health, my life, and I can't get it back)?"

Confronting "What's the Use?" Thinking

Let's look at this problem from a different angle, and see how guilt and shame fuel "What's the use?" thinking and its **hidden expectation of perfection**.

While guilt is associated with something we've done or should have done, shame is about who we are deep inside. *Shame is a deep sense of inferiority and unworthiness that we feel others can see, and that we can't get rid of or change.* This will sometimes result in feelings of humiliation or extreme embarrassment, as well as the urge to run and hide. We can't move forward to figure out new ways of tackling a problem because we're convinced there is nothing that can change the way we feel and think about ourselves. In essence, our thinking gets stuck on "What's the use?" ("…because I am that bad, sick, or broken, and this whole situation is hopeless.")

In shame we see a deeper, more ingrained level of the more common inadequacies we all feel sometimes when we compare ourselves to others, or how we should be according to our internal (learnt and often unspoken) expectations of ourselves. While guilt can spur us onward to do something different, shame does not give us any wiggle room. With shame, we feel we must meet our (unrealistic) standards and expectations or we feel we are abject failures. There is a hidden perfectionism at work that says the person has to be perfect, as well as "good" and deserving of love and success (good things or rewards for my actions, including a quick return to health).

The counterpoints to shame and its perfectionism is *self-acceptance* and *self-compassion*. This is where we have a realistic sense of what human nature is like, and what is possible in life and with ourselves. Thus we accept our gifts and strengths, as well as acknowledge and accept our weaknesses, mistakes, and failures, including aging, physical decline, and illness.

After all, we know we all fail in some way, sometime – it's the nature of life – and we all make mistakes, big and small. If we can accept this fundamental truth, we can be kind to ourselves – and from that flows kindness and acceptance towards others as well. There is no shame in imperfection, for that is the nature of being human.

When those in rehab exhibit shame's underlying perfectionism, I sometimes use a sports analogy to change their unrealistic expectations. In baseball, for example, a player can get into the Hall of Fame and be considered a great player if they bat .300. That hitting percentage indicates they struck out, or did not make a hit, 70 percent of the time! In other words, they failed and made *mistakes most of the time, and yet are still great Hall of Famers*. In tennis the percentage is much higher because of the nature of the game, but not even the greatest tennis players win 100 percent of the time. This is true for any sport – as well as the arts, medicine, research, and all other areas of life.

Perfection does not happen. It cannot happen. It's not in the nature of our humanity. As a result, I'll ask the resident, "Why do you have to 'bat a thousand' when no one else does or can?" (If you've never heard the old saying "batting a thousand" or 1.000 percent, it means absolutely no mistakes or failures. The baseball player makes a hit every time, the tennis player wins every game and match, the golfer makes a birdie or better on every hole, and so on.)

The resident doesn't have an answer to my question, of course. No one does. What was operating was their old childhood programming: It was rearing its head and showing us what their parents and teachers wanted in order to be approved of, rewarded, and loved. I ask the question not get an answer, but to jog the old perfectionistic programming loose from its moorings to make room for the energy of a new idea to seep in.

Then I always add, "In rehab no one does it 100 percent right, 100 percent of the time, and no one improves daily. This does not happen, cannot happen."

Interestingly, some residents actually balk at this idea. Their old programming is so entrenched they can't imagine questioning it, much less thinking or doing something different.

"What's the use?" thinking harbors similar unrealistic expectations that center on the idea, "I should be getting better according to my timetable and my standards, and if I'm not, then it's not worth working so hard because I'll never get what I want (and go home)." What the resident doesn't yet understand is that rehab is a roller-coaster ride with "good days" and "bad days." But with determined "right" effort over time, they increase their chances of regaining their functioning and independence, and going home which is what they all want.

> If you want to experience fear…get a future. If you want to experience shame and guilt, get a past. If you want to experience peace, discover who you are without your story.
> ~ Byron Katie

Handling the Ups and Downs

A simple, straightforward approach to rehab works best. The focus needs to be on the essentials and anything that can't wait.

Residents worry and fret about all sorts of things – some incredibly minor items that have nothing to do with rehab or their discharge, or perhaps things they can do nothing about. For that reason, I recommend residents do the following *every single day of their rehab to optimize their recovery and go home as soon as possible.*

First and foremost, residents in rehab need to *keep their focus on today and only today – this present moment.* This means using the well-known **"one day at a time"** approach.

For most people this is easier said than done. The mind will put out all sorts of protests why this is not possible. For example, people may claim it's "stupid," or, "too hard," or, "won't work" – so "why try it?"

Don't give in to this mind chatter. The mind likes to chew on complexity and dualities, often creating complication when none actually exists. An antidote to this internal chatter is to emphasize that if others can be successful in rehab and use a "one day at a time" approach, why can't you?

The mind also likes to be in one of two places: in the future or in the past. Staying present, today, in this moment, is initially challenging. One quick and effective way to return to the present moment when you're stewing over something and getting nowhere is to ask yourself:

What do I need to do *right now*?

You'll find that the answer is usually, "Nothing; not a thing." Or else, the answer will be simple and straightforward, such as, "I need to go to physical therapy, shower, eat lunch, call my daughter for some clothes, pay the electric bill," and so on. If, for example, you need to pay bills, then do so and *return your focus to your rehab*. Don't waste precious energy ruminating about the stack of bills piling up at home and then do nothing about it.

Second, rehab will be up and down, like a roller-coaster. Rehab, or any medical recovery or sports training, is never a straight line upwards despite what we want or expect of ourselves and our bodies. Up and down means just that: There will be "good days," and there will be "bad days." It happens to everybody, and more than once.

What's more, a bad day can happen after a good day. For instance, a resident will report they're finally feeling good and walked a hundred feet in therapy, and that tomorrow they're going to walk two hundred feet. What happens tomorrow? They can't get out of bed, everything hurts, and they can't imagine doing therapy, much less walking anywhere.

When a bad day comes along, the challenge is not to get discouraged and give up. The simple thing to do is *to realize what's happening and remind yourself, "It's a bad day," and move forward*. That means doing whatever therapy is possible — even if it's light – and moving forward by doing rehab's two main jobs.

Doing Rehab "Right"

Residents have two **jobs to do every day** – and only two – in order to do rehab right to optimize their recovery and get home. If I ask them what they think these jobs are, they'll usually answer "Get better" or something similar.

I respond, "No, that's not it. Think again, what do you think might be your number one job here?"

They're stumped. Are you wondering why "Get better" isn't the primary job? Well, it's too broad and vague; no one actually knows what "get better" means or how to get there. As a result, it will not guide them to their rehab goals. So I've made rehab's two jobs simple and concrete so there's no ambiguity.

The two rehab jobs are:

• **Job #1: Do therapy every day**, unless there's significant illness or pain. **This is the most important thing a rehab resident will do to get themselves ready to go home.** If they're hurting or sick, the resident (or their family) needs to discuss it with their therapist, nurse and/or physician or surgeon. Importantly, therapy works best with consistency and repetition, slowly increasing difficulty over time. A little here, a little there, will not accomplish anything.

Some residents believe it's up to them when they'll do therapy, saying they'll do therapy when they feel better – e.g., tomorrow or next week, or when they feel like it. Of course residents have the legal right to say, "No" to any therapy or treatment, but this is not what is happening here. Rather, these residents have the misguided notion that therapy is optional and not particularly important to their recovery. What they fail to recognize is that everything medically can go right and they recover from their illness or surgery, *but if they don't recover their functioning to do the basic requirements of daily life, their independence is at risk.*

Residents need to work with their therapists, forging an effective partnership. However, sometimes the resident and therapist mix about as well as oil and water. If the resident does not like their assigned therapist or can't seem to communicate well with them, request a change. The goal is to have a good rehab, not to make friends or avoid hurting someone feelings. There's work to be done if they want to recover and go home, and that needs to be the priority.

Sometimes new residents do not understand what their therapy can gift them with, and tell me it is "silly," "stupid," "boring," and/or "repetitive." This is more frequently expressed by those having Speech Therapy, since some residents do not like the cognitive exercises, believing these are beneath them. I remind these residents that each therapy exercise has a purpose: *Physical* for the waist down and walking; *Occupational* for upper body strength we need every day and to get up from a chair, etc., and *Speech* for speaking, swallowing, and cognition. Each exercise is focused on different muscles or processes. In addition, the brain/mind needs to be exercised as much as the body. As a result, there is no such thing as a "silly" or "useless" rehab exercise.

Furthermore, whatever therapy regime is instituted, it is the one the resident needs for their medical problems based on various medical assessments, and this could well include cognitive and memory exercises. Sure, not every resident gets assigned to do them, but that's because not everyone needs them. So if you're assigned cognitive exercises, do them diligently, hopefully with a smile because it'll make it easier and go faster. Remember, the goal is to get healthier and stronger in order to go home.

- **Job #2: Take care of the Basics: Eat, Drink Water, and Rest.**

As mentioned previously, it's essential the basics are taken care of in order to pave the road for a better, quicker recovery. That means eat enough and well enough for the body to recover and have energy for rehab.

Drink plenty of water, if not on fluid restriction. Please note this does not include soft drinks, iced tea, coffee, or juice all day long. The body needs *water*, not repeat doses of sugar and caffeine.

Rest. This does not necessarily mean sleep eight hours total, or an all-night sleep. Rest, and even take naps as long as they're not too late in the day to interfere with nighttime sleep. Avoid stimulants like coffee, tea, or colas after six p.m. Steer clear from energy drinks (too much caffeine) or sport drinks (too much sugar). Avoid drinking lots of water in the evening since that will mean trips to the bathroom in the middle of the night, as well as waiting for assistance to help you to the bathroom. If you can't seem to sleep, tell your nurse. Also, do the 4 - 4 breathing to help your mind calm down so you can fall asleep.

If the resident's spouse is still alive and involved, they also need to pay attention to these Basics themselves. Some spouses spend a great deal of time in the facility, and over time this schedule and their stress and worry will wear them out. After all, they are not twenty-one anymore and don't have the reserves they once had. And if they don't take care of the Basics for themselves, their health will be at risk, especially since many already have chronic health conditions.

For the elderly spouse, this self-care means adding one additional activity and that is: *daily exercise to help get rid of stress*. This can be as easy as walking the mall or the neighborhood. In short, *do anything that moves the body*. Other valuable activities include lunch with friends, engaging in a hobby or favorite pastime, and attending a support group related to their resident's condition, such as a dementia support group. Any down time or self-nourishing activity the spouse engages in helps maintain their own health.

We often tend to bypass the Basics, thinking they are not particularly important. But these Basics set the foundation for healthy living and recovery for our loved one as well as ourselves.

Sometimes I'll add another job to the resident's and spouse's list and that is the all-important…**Breathe**. Breathe slowly and gently to the belly button, exhaling long into a sigh. Repeat three times in a row. Do this as often as you can remember.

> Live as if you were to die tomorrow.
> Learn as if you were to live forever.
> ~ Mahatma Gandhi

Turtle Time

The old children's story of the race between the tortoise and the hare illustrates another important point regarding how to manage a rehab stay effectively.

In the story, the rabbit takes off leaving the turtle far behind. The rabbit, however, gets bored and starts to go here and there, losing his focus and his goal, which was to win the race. The turtle keeps plodding along, putting one stumpy leg in front of the other, the spotlight firmly fixed on the end point.

Who won the race? The slow and steady turtle.

And the rabbit? Who knows where he went as he dashed off into the landscapes of a wandering mind?

Rehab is "turtle time." Everybody wants to speed rehab up and get home, but they don't know how to do that because it cannot be done. The body heals in its own way and in its own time.

If you find yourself in rehab, be a turtle. Slow and steady wins this race.

Leaving "AMA"

"AMA" means "Against Medical Advice" and signifies that a rehab resident has decided to leave the facility before they have completed their rehab and sign themselves out.

Such a decision happens infrequently, but when it does the resident usually has gone down this route because they are angry about being confined and resent all the facility's rules and regulations. Commonly they present a laundry list of complaints that simply cannot be remedied.

Most importantly, such residents are in pervasive denial of their medical status; what they need to do to recover and effectively manage their illness; and what they need to be able to do to live independently. They want to go home and they want it now – and they will not listen to anyone. Although they usually get some assistance from a family member or friend, this is someone who also doesn't seem to understand the seriousness of the situation and/or has their own agenda.

For example, one senior who left AMA denied she had a major colon infection (C. Diff or Clostridium difficile), saying her test results were "normal" when they were not. She insisted she could recuperate as well at home (a common belief). After all, she claimed, "No one at the nursing home ever checked on [her] or helped anyway," and, "The nurses didn't know how to do medications," and, the food she was given was "slop," and her room was "never cleaned." On and on and on it went. So, while her husband was of town, she called her grandson and told him to take her home.

She lasted three days at home before uncontrollably high sugar levels landed her back in the hospital, and then back in rehab. Hopefully, she finally learned to do rehab right and avoid unnecessary medical complications.

Another resident, a skinny eighty-nine-year-old man with a pelvic fracture, denied his fragile condition, even though it took two therapists to help him walk ten feet after a month in rehab. (Pelvic fractures take a long time to heal, and a month is only the beginning.) But he wanted to go home *now*. His wife (age eighty-seven and with mild cognitive impairment and other health issues) wanted him home *now* as well. In fact, she repeated this desire every day, even asking if she could take him out to a restaurant for lunch.

But she didn't have an answer when I asked her how she was going to get him in and out of the car when he couldn't get out of bed by himself and she didn't have the strength to help him. She wasn't even considering the pain a new pelvic fracture gives with any movement. Both were also opposed to their children's plan to move them back north to be near them, saying they "loved" their retirement home and "didn't need help."

So, at the one-month mark, this resident figured that since he was now in less pain and could stand (true) and "walk" (ten feet with help), he was ready to go home. Somehow he convinced his orthopedist to release him from rehab with (limited) home health services. This was not AMA, but close to it since no one in the rehab center, including the Medical Director, thought he was ready. The man died less than two months later after another hospitalization.

When these types of situations arise, there is almost nothing the family, facility, or medical staff can do. These residents have made up their mind, and denied and rationalized away the extent of their medical crisis and infirmity. They also have the legal right to leave if they are competent and do not pose a danger to themselves to the point the State can intervene. In these circumstances, a family can only wait helplessly on the sidelines until a catastrophe develops – and it will, sooner or later. Only then will their loved one allow guidance and assistance.

As I sometimes remind upset families and staff, these residents, like everybody else have the right to make decisions, even "bad" or unhealthy decisions. We cannot save them from themselves; that's their job.

> I long, as does every human being,
> to be at home wherever I find myself.
> ~ Maya Angelou

"When Do I Get Out of Here?"

Residents often ask me who decides when they can go home, and why don't they have a date yet. I explain to them in basic terms that upon their admission, there is an overall sense of what they need to be able to do, given their medical situation, in order to go home safely. For example, with a knee or hip replacement the most basic goal is for the resident to be able to get out of bed or a chair and walk a reasonable distance. The staff and attending physician do not have a specific discharge date even though they know more or less how long it should take, assuming no complications. Once again, we must always keep age, general health, and complications in mind.

As the resident progresses in rehab, the rehab therapists keep track of their progress and will report and make recommendations to the attending physician and/or surgeon. Once the resident is nearing their rehab goals, they project a discharge date. The Medical Director of the facility and/or the surgeon will review and approve or change this projected date. If the resident wants to know how they are doing and what progress they have made, their best source of information is their rehab therapists since they can describe it in detail based on their assessments.

Once a discharge date is recommended and a Home Evaluation is (usually) completed, the social worker or discharge planner takes care of the details, including coordinating with family or other responsible individuals such as a Legal Guardian. This is a basic outline of what happens in a Florida skilled nursing rehab facility.

Providing this basic information is generally enough for most rehab residents to "get the picture," as well as remind them of what other staff has already told them which they often didn't completely understand, remember, or trust. In addition, I always remind the resident that neither the facility nor their insurance and other third party payers such as Medicare want them to stay long-term. The facility's goal is for a "good" rehab – and then send them home. This is important to emphasize since many rehab residents fear that they are going to be locked up in a nursing home forever.

Sometimes it becomes clear that a resident cannot return home, either because of a health decline and/or inability to progress enough in rehab to master the skills necessary to live independently. As a result, they may need to go into a semi-independent Assisted Living Facility (ALF) or into Long-Term Care in a nursing home. No one, no matter what their age or condition is expecting this outcome.

At times, family members want to tell the resident that an ALF or Long-Term Care is the plan as soon as it's decided – which could be weeks before their rehab discharge. I recommend against this course of action unless it's close to the end of the resident's rehab. Why? It's simple, actually: If we tell the resident this plan and they still have a way to go in their rehab, their disappointment in not going home can easily interfere with rehab. For example, they may well give up or put out little effort, not appreciating what rehab can still do for them even if they are not going home.

Since the goal is to get residents as strong and as functional as possible regardless of their placement, I recommend they not be told they are not going home for the time being and that everyone continue to encourage rehab. There will be time enough later to discuss transferring to an ALF or long-term care, but not now. It's not needed. That said, in a few instances the resident recognizes they cannot live alone or in the home of their son or daughter, and having adjusted well to the nursing home, they actually are relieved when told of a discharge placement into an ALF or to long-term nursing home care.

How to tell someone they're not going home and are going into an ALF or nursing home long-term will be covered in Chapter 6. For now, let's move forward to the going home process.

You Can't Make Someone Happy

Lovely Eunice was ninety-three and ready to go home. She had successfully completed a long rehab stay for a cardiac condition and pneumonia. You'd think Eunice would be happy, but that was far from her reality. She wanted to stay in the nursing home, *but* hated the food because it wasn't like what she was used to. She was offered an ALF most people would envy, *but* she refused to consider it. Her only daughter wanted Eunice to move north so she would be near family and not alone in Florida, *but* Eunice also said "No" to this option. Eunice's daughter, at wit's end and needing to return home, arranged for live-in help that Eunice also didn't want.

I asked Eunice, who was in an obvious funk, what the problem was.

"I'm stubborn. I always have been," she answered with a shrug.

I tried a few interventions, but Eunice was having nothing of it. She was stuck in a long-standing unhappiness of her own making. She probably was past the point where she could make meaningful changes to her rigid expectations of how life should be. There was no negotiating or problem solving with Eunice because she refused on principle. Her stubbornness had won the day – but would bring her and her daughter needless misery.

What else could her daughter have done? Not much.

You can't make someone else happy or satisfied with life, much less cooperate or adapt to health and lifestyle changes. That's *their* job. A caregiver sometimes has to accept a loved one's "bad" choices, and then wait for the catastrophe or crisis that will surely come and opens the door to greater assistance.

In all probability Eunice will end up in long-term care sooner rather than later, but of course not in a nursing home she would like or approve of, and certainly not one that would suit her culinary standards. A lifetime of stubborn and inflexible choices and expectations was leading her down that unhappy road as much as old age.

> When you drop your expectations that a person, a situation, a place, or an object should fulfill you, it's easier to be present in this moment because you're no longer looking to the next one. Most people want to get what they want, whereas the secret is to want what you get at this moment.
> ~ Eckhart Tolle

Going Home

It's not unusual for a resident to feel anxious or even worried about going home. It may have been weeks, or even months, since they were home, and without any awareness they have grown accustomed to having others around them who help with everyday tasks and make recovery easier. Moreover, the resident may be worried whether to not they can take care of what they need to do at home.

For example, what if they won't able to pick up things from the floor or from high places, do laundry, get groceries, cook, clean the house, manage their medications and doctors' appointments, dress and shower on their own? Or, if they live with someone, how will they fare when the adult child they live with is at work? If they still live with an elderly spouse, what happens if the spouse they depend on becomes sick and incapacitated? Adding to the catalog of these common concerns and "What ifs," is that some residents might also miss the nursing home staff they have come to know, and which relieved the loneliness they felt back home where they lived alone.

As you see from this list of worries, residents can easily get tangled in a spider's web of "What if…?" thinking. Yes, all their concerns may revolve about practical matters and chores, and indeed it will be necessary to manage them at some point. But, no one cannot resolve a vague "What if?" that resides somewhere in the future. At best, we can use a "What if?" in order to plan a strategy or take preliminary steps toward resolving a problem if it actually occurs.

However, in my experience, a "What if…?" is not a call to practical planning, but the mind spinning itself into a spider web of anxieties and fear. Thus, **the first step is help the resident return to the present moment by asking: "What needs to be done now? What's the first step that needs to be taken now?"**

> A journey of a thousand miles must begin with a single step.
> ~ Lao-Tze

Going home usually involves getting basic questions answered by the social worker or discharge planner. These may include: "Will I get a walker or do I have to buy one? How will I continue my therapy? Do I leave the facility with medications?"

The initial answer to these questions is that the nursing home staff will discuss these and other discharge considerations with the resident and/or their family member, as well as arrange any required medical equipment and services.

The second step is to acknowledge the anxieties, worries, and even fears. Ask your loved one what are they worried about. Then, make a list of their worries and fears. Once the list is complied, remind the resident that they have been doing many of their daily tasks in the facility. Moreover, the way to continue building their skills is to follow what they have been taught in a step-wise fashion. These include how to get in and out of a car, walk up steps, walk upright and heel-toe, shower, etc.

Bear in mind, however, that people make **two primary mistakes** when they go home. These two mistakes are actually two sides of the same coin.

• Mistake #1: Doing too much, too fast, too soon.

Rather than bypassing this important point by assuming you know what it means, take a moment to read it again and reflect what it means. Also, figure out how it applies to the resident's life (or your own even if you're not about to be discharged from rehab).

Doing too much – too many steps or activities in a row for a still weak body or body part

Too fast – going too quickly for a body that is still recovering

Too soon – the body simply isn't ready yet ("…But I'm going to do it anyway because I've always done it.")

One woman in her early seventies went home after a successful rehab, and the very next week went into her kitchen to make lunch. She had three things she wanted to do: put her groceries away, make a sandwich, and clean up the counter before she sat down to her lunch. She put away the groceries, but when she started making the sandwich, she felt very tired. She finished the sandwich and walked toward the refrigerator, and felt a stab of pain in her new hip. Then in the next instant, she fell and broke her hip…again. Her mistake was not listening to her body when she first felt tired and then changing her priorities.

Pain or feeling tired is the body's way of telling you to stop. LISTEN to it: Sit down and rest! The sandwich will still be here, the counter can be cleaned anytime, and whatever else needs to be done can wait. This woman didn't stop and ended up in surgery for another hip replacement, and another more complicated rehab stay.

Just because someone completes rehab does not mean their body is fully recovered. For instance, doctors say a knee replacement will take about twelve months to completely heal while bilateral knee replacements take eighteen to twenty-four months.

Next, let me bring up a common situation that becomes a challenge as we age. An elderly man wakes up in the middle of the night to go to the bathroom. He decided not to turn on the light or use the new walker he received from the rehab center, thinking, "It's only a few feet (to my *ensuite* bathroom). I don't really need it."

What happened? He fell in the dark bathroom, hit his head, and broke his leg. He didn't have a phone or a medical alert device on him, so he spent a few painful hours on the floor until his son found him the next day.

The Centers for Disease Control and Prevention (CDC) reports in "Older Adult Falls" that each year one out of three elderly adults (age sixty-five and up) falls, *with less than half of those telling their doctors of the incident*. This means that every year millions of seniors fall, and over 700,000 are hospitalized, primarily for broken hips or head injuries.

From what residents have told me through the years, most falls happen in the early morning hours when they are going to the bathroom. It's probably because we're half asleep and not paying attention to what we're doing. Plus, we need to urinate quickly, and so proceed by habit. After all, since early childhood we've been getting up and going to the bathroom whenever we like without having to think about any of the steps involved. In old age we continue this habit, forgetting our body has changed – usually a lot more than we realize.

Falls often result in serious consequences for the older adult. And so, in our senior years, we need to develop new habits with new steps that require us to think about what we're going to do before we do it in order to do it safely.

Here's another example to drive this important point home. An elderly couple who had been in rehab together for separate aliments insisted on going home before the attending physician and rehab therapists thought they were ready. A week later, the still weak husband tried to help his wife, who could barely walk, get out of bed one morning. They both fell to the floor and ended up in the hospital, one needing surgery, both needing rehab and later long-term care.

On the other side of the coin lies the second mistake.

• Mistake #2: Doing too little.

Residents are so glad be back home and not "have to do" rehab, that they sit and become the proverbial "couch potatoes." Instead of doing their therapy exercises regularly, they embody attitudes along the lines of, "Not today," or, "I'm too busy and don't have time," or, "I don't feel like it," or, "It's getting late. I'll do it tomorrow." And so on. But tomorrow isn't a good day either…and then they haven't done their exercises in months.

All this time they're getting weaker and still believe they're fine until the day comes when they fall again or can't climb up the stairs or get off the toilet.

This happens more often than anyone likes to admit.

The moral of this story is do your *physical therapy exercises regularly even if you've gone home*. The human body was meant to move. The older we get, the more we need to exercise it in order to maintain our functioning level and independence. Don't be like one long-term care resident who reported that one morning she woke up and tried to get out of bed, but her legs wouldn't move. And they never did again, despite repeat courses of physical therapy that could not strengthen her long underused and weak muscles. Her legs had retired permanently on her, as they often do on many of us.

>Aging is not lost youth
>but a new stage of opportunity and strength.
>~ Betty Friedan

Time-Tested Tips

- Listen to your loved one and they'll let you know what's on their mind. If they express some version of "What the use?" or "Why bother?" don't try to talk them out of how they feel, just listen. It is not your job to be their psychotherapist, or figure out how to make their rehab enjoyable or successful. However, do ask simply worded, basic questions to find out how they feel or what they're worried about. And, request mental health services if their mood or attitude is hindering their rehab participation.

- Rehab involves taking a day-to-day approach and doing two basic jobs. What are they?

- Going Home brings up two common mistakes. What are they? Recognize they apply to all of us as we get older, even if we never go into rehab.

- **Practice 4 - 4 Breathing:** Breathe in slowly and gently to a count of 4.
  Imagine your breath going all the way down to your belly button.
  Then purse your lips and exhale slowly and gently for a count of 4.
  Imagine your breath flowing outward like a soft breeze, leaving in its wake an alert mind and a relaxed, alive body.

GETTING OLDER BEING HERE

At fifteen, my heart was set on learning.
At thirty, I stood firm.
At forty, I had no more doubts.
At fifty, I knew the will of heaven.
At sixty, my ear was obedient.
At seventy, I could follow my heart's desire without overstepping the bounds of what was right.
~ Confucius

Chapter 5
What Would You Do?

Supporting and advocating for your loved one in rehab is both more complicated and delicate than it first appears. What exactly does support and encouragement mean? Should you push them or stand back, and perhaps watch them fail and never get the chance to return home again? When do we need to take an active, even assertive role on their behalf? And when are we meddling or trying to advance our own agenda instead of advocating wisely for a loved one? Below we'll explore some of these issues and choices, ending with an example that'll ask you to decide, "What would you do?"

The Drill Sergeant

A common mistake spouses and adult children make when trying to encourage their loved one is to nag, scold, badger, criticize, bully, and repeat what the patient needs to do over and over again. Family members have said they, "…must do this or their loved one will not progress," often using the "No pain, no gain" motto of a famous sports commercial. But rehab is *not* sports training, and even in sports, constant badgering is counterproductive and sabotages self-esteem and focus. In addition, these residents are not young and healthy athletes in training for a competition, and family are not professional trainers.

This is the Drill Sergeant approach, and *it does not work*. If they are on the receiving end of this approach, the resident may shut down or even refuse therapy, 'digging in their heels' because they don't like being told what to do by a wife or husband, much less an adult child they once wiped clean. They may also feel no one is listening to them or considering their needs in this painful, confusing, and scary situation. It's *nag, nag, nag*, and no one likes it or responds well to it.

I recommend to families that they retire from their Drill Sergeant job: It's stressful for them as well as the resident. I also explain to them that the staff does enough in terms of "getting after" the residents.

In addition, the resident may listen more to me, the psychologist, as a healthcare professional than to family members whom the resident probably has been tuning out on some level for years. The resident may also respect recommendations from a professional more because in their eyes it carries more weight or substance.

Besides, a family member cannot effectively reframe and guide them as to what they need to do in rehab when it's not their field of expertise and training.

It's also important to remember, however, that the resident does have the legal right to refuse therapy and treatments. And if they do, the staff is legally obligated to respect that choice. After all, the resident like everyone else has the right to make choices – even bad ones. They also might not be able to physically or mentally do what we are expecting and asking them to do.

The Meddlers

From time to time I'll see family members attend therapy sessions with their resident. They believe that in doing so they're encouraging their loved one, supporting them through a difficult time. Therapists on the other hand are uniformly polite and so generally will not tell family not to attend. However, in my view, *you should not attend therapy with your resident unless the therapist has asked you to attend for a specific reason.*

It's important to remember that all residents have less than their normal amount of energy and concentration, and as we age, our ability to multi-task decreases. As a result, a family's presence in therapy will divert the resident's energy and focus, as well as that of other rehab residents since therapy usually occurs in a large room with as many as a dozen or more residents and staff present. Consequently, all the other sick and infirmed residents often end up watching your family and not listening to their own therapist.

Here's a real life example to highlight the problem. A ninety-year-old frail man came into rehab with a large New York City Italian family that hovered over him. These family members would tell him to eat, drink his protein shake, sit, stand up, put his leg into his pant leg or move his arm back whenever the aide was trying to dress him, and so on. This continued on into the therapy room where at times several family members surrounded him, along with his therapist and eight to twelve other residents and therapists in the room. This resident would aimlessly look from one of his loved ones to the other, seldom following what his therapist told him to do, seemingly lost in all the words and commands coming at him.

I suggested to this family they refrain from going into the therapy room and allow him to work with his therapist on his own. They outright refused. His daughter said this was their heritage and they were there to help him. The poor fellow never progressed and went into long-term care as weak as the day he was brought in from the hospital.

Long-term care had become inevitable for this resident: What this family had not seen was that they were "helping" him out of their own anxiety and emotional needs. They repeatedly stepped into the role of therapist and aide even though they were untrained and unqualified for the job. They wanted "Daddy" to get better and believed they themselves had to actively direct and cajole him to get there. In blindly following their family programming of what a supportive and loving family does, and dismissing what trained professionals recommended, this family lost sight of what their loved one needed to support his rehab and maximize his recovery.

When my own father was in rehab, I encouraged and supported him by wishing him a good therapy session, *and then I left*. My dad loved therapy and went from falling repeatedly and confined to a wheel-chair to walking hundreds of feet with a walker (something he would continue to do for several years). He ended up in long-term care, but it wasn't because of lack of therapy effort or progress, or my meddling in his rehab therapies.

> To change the world, we must be good to those who cannot repay us.
> ~ Pope Francis

Effective Advocates

Attempting to support a loved one in rehab may involve needing to be their advocate, and this typically requires having the legal right to do so. Healthcare advocacy means speaking on behalf of the resident, especially one that cannot speak for themselves due to age, illness, or dementia. The basic goal is to ensure the resident gets the medical care they need, including providing information, coordinating services to support and help improve their health, and safeguarding their rights and privacy.

Advocacy is a nuanced skill that involves many factors and is not a straight forward proposition as those on the outside of the situation sometimes think. As a result, well-meaning friends and relatives sometimes offer uninformed and unwise advice. There are also legal issues we must be mindful of at every turn. Advocacy will also change over time as our loved one's age, condition, and circumstances shift and new priorities emerge.

It's important to remember your adult, legally competent loved one who is now in rehab has the right to make medical decisions, including the right to refuse services and treatments. You cannot save them from themselves and their "bad" or wrong choices. And if you try to impose your preferences or what you think they should do, it will make a difficult situation even more stressful and contentious for all concerned. Let me share with you an example of **runaway advocacy,** where a family member lost sight of the resident and her wishes.

Joan, age ninety-three, came into rehab with multiple health problems and could only do a limited rehab. Although disappointed, Joan accepted the fact her health was failing and she needed long-term care. Her oldest daughter, Emily, did not. She often appeared frantic and kept insisting that the nursing home "do more" in order to get her mother well and return home. At one point, Emily announced, "I always fix things."

"Some things are not fixable," I gently corrected her.

"I'll fix this," she rebutted, and strode down the hall, a new list of demands in hand. Essentially, she wanted more rehab for her mother even though Joan physically could not do the exercises and was in a lot of pain. Emily's brothers tried to explain their mother was failing and in pain, but still she refused to listen. To make a long story short, Joan's health continued to deteriorate, and her daughter somehow engineered a transfer to inpatient rehab followed by another admission to skilled nursing rehab where Joan made even less progress.

By this point, Joan was at peace with her decline, and even looked forward to death since she had no illusions as to her condition. She even told me during her second rehab she wished her daughter would stop her bossy meddling and just, "…let her be." But when I asked her if she'd told her daughter how she felt, Joan simply said, "No. She'll do what she wants." And she did, until finally Joan went into hospice care and died a week later.

It can be said that runaway advocacy comes from love and the desire not to lose our loved one, but we always need to ask: What does the resident want? What's in *their* best interest?

For example, a frail hundred-year-old man came into rehab with a feeding tube (stressful for someone this age). He could barely do any rehab or talk. Yet his only daughter Gretchen (in her mid-seventies) demanded he be taken to various activities to give him more social contact and intellectual stimulation.

Activities in a skilled nursing home are primarily for long-term residents since rehab residents need *all* their energy for rehab and recovery. By and large rehab residents do not attend activities until they are well along their rehab and feeling much better, with extra energy for these type of social activities. In this case, Gretchen would not accept her father was near the end of his life and proceeded from that belief, demanding social activities that were both taxing and inappropriate for him. This man died late one night a few days later.

> When you say or do anything to please, get, keep,
> influence, or control anyone or anything, fear is the
> cause and pain is the result.
> ~ Byron Katie

Below I'll use my husband's double knee replacement surgery and rehab as an example of **advocacy issues that can come up with a more alert, and somewhat younger, resident**. Then I'll use my then eighty-year-old father's medical crisis, hospitalization, and rehab as an example of issues and choices that can arise with an older parent's decline.

Advocating for an Alert, 'Younger' Resident

When he was in his late sixties, my husband, Norman, underwent bilateral knee replacement surgery. This involves a painful recovery, and can take up to two years for a full recovery. Prior to this surgery, Norman and I took the necessary steps that gave me the legal authority to access his medical records, speak with his medical provides, and make medical and financial decisions if he was incapable of doing so. Together the two of us also discussed his wishes, including worst-case scenarios, and which skilled nursing rehab center he would go into. I gave Norman two choices of facilities I'd worked in for years and felt confident he would receive good nursing care and rehab therapy in either one.

After receiving double knee replacements, a patient often needs to be in a rehab facility, and this came to pass with Norman. After surgery, Norman could not stand without almost fainting (due to falling blood pressure), much less walk the required distance (about seventy-five feet) in order to be discharged home.

In addition, following his surgery and while still in the hospital, Norman lost a great deal of blood, necessitating two units of blood and an extra day in the hospital. And of course, he needed and received large doses of pain medication. Because of his age, mental competency, and his long-standing relationship with his orthopedist, I was never consulted in the medical decision-making while he was in the hospital. Rather, Norman made all decisions even though he was often more than a little out it and his memory was spotty. I did not agree with this process, but I had no choice but to accept it. If Norman's condition had worsened, my advocacy role would definitely have changed and I would have taken charge. Thus, my only role while Norman was in the hospital was to take care of minor issues with the nursing staff and support him as best I could. I did make it a point to check in with the nurses every day, and for every shift, so I knew what was happening and they knew Norman was not entirely on his own.

When it came time for Norman's discharge to the rehab facility, I became actively involved since the hospital had not input his discharge into their computer system, and the hospital's discharge department was not returning my or the nurse's calls. So I took matters into my own hands and called the nursing home's Admissions Director, since they need to be alerted of pending discharges to prepare for the resident's arrival. I asked her for assistance since the hospital was not cooperating. The Admissions Director came through, and Norman was finally transferred to the nursing home that evening. That was how I served as my husband's advocate for his hospital stay.

Once Norman was in the nursing home I became more active since I knew the staff and the rehab process. I made sure to receive daily updates, including his medications and his dips in blood pressure, which now resulted in his therapy being stopped mid-session, which was not a good development. I had no contact with the orthopedist, who never called me, but I spoke regularly with the in-house Medical Director in charge of my husband's daily care. He soon asked the consulting cardiologist to evaluate Norman, and that doctor determined the problem was resulting from his high dosage of pain medication. Once the medication problem was resolved, Norman's rehab took off and he was able to go home in four weeks.

I already knew the pain medication was the problem, but it's always best if the doctors are primary in making medical recommendations. Sometimes family members demand certain medications and/or medical treatments, but this can result in unnecessary problems and power struggles. I believe it's more effective to form a partnership with the medical staff, rather than dictate care when I lack the necessary expertise.

In sum: When supporting and advocating for a more alert resident, family members typically should take a back seat

and follow the resident's lead, unless there is an emergency or a serious issue (like the one my husband faced).

> Do what you can, with what you have, where you are.
> ~ Theodore Roosevelt

Advocating for an Elderly Parent, Spouse, Sibling, or Partner

When advocating for someone who is elderly, the advocacy role can be very different as well as more challenging, especially since it will trigger your early emotional programming.

My independent and prideful Cuban father lived alone across the state, and a four-hour drive away from me. For years I was able to do little aside from gently and repeatedly suggesting he move to where I lived so he would have support close by as he grew older. Preferring to be in control of his life, my father would have nothing of this advice. But when he stopped returning my phone calls, I decided it was time to see him in person. I finally got lucky when he answered his phone and I could make a date.

What I found when my husband and I arrived at my father's condo shocked me. The apartment was not as clean and tidy as it had always been. Nor had my father remembered we were coming for a Thanksgiving visit. He was not mentally alert, and talked less than usual. In fact, he seemed to be in mid-to-late stage dementia, and had difficulty putting on his trousers so we could go out as we had planned. When we finally went outside his home, he also walked so slowly and precariously my husband had to hold his arm.

When I asked about his current health, he denied having any problems, his pride and independent streak still intact.

Although I had no legal permission in hand to obtain any of my father's medical information from his long-term primary care doctor, I nevertheless wrote his physician. I described what I found in detail, and requested an immediate referral for physical therapy since I was concerned my father would fall and break a hip. Actually he'd already fallen, but never told me when it happened, and he probably never told his doctor like the majority of seniors fail to.

I later found out my father never showed up for the physical therapy evaluation because he forgot he had an appointment. Due to confidentially laws, I never received a response from his primary care doctor. I don't know whether the doctor's office never asked him for next-of-kin information and permission as they probably should have with an elderly patient, or whether they were being negligent.

My hands were tied: This was all I could do for my father at that time since he denied any problems and was rebuffing my assistance at every turn. The reality is, there is little a family member can do unless the senior is in danger and the State's Adult Protective Services or similar agency can be called in. My father was not at that point, so I knew I had to wait until a crisis erupted before I could do more. I've heard similar stories many times over in my nursing home career, and I've counseled many about the need to sit and wait, for they will be needed later.

About month later, my father called and said he was ready to move to be near me. I told him I would start making arrangements.

Just a few days later I received a call from my uncle who said a Daytona Beach hospital had called him about my father. I found out that my father had driven himself to the hospital near his condo, only to discover he could not walk the distance to the emergency entrance. He had to hug a light pole to avoid falling. Thankfully, a security guard saw him and alerted emergency personnel.

Even though my father had my business card in his wallet and we share the same surname, the hospital never thought to call me. Somehow though, they managed to track down my uncle several hundred miles away. When I called the hospital and informed them I was next of kin, I did get some preliminary medical information, but the hospital refused to give me more than that. Nonetheless, I began making arrangements to transfer my father to a rehab facility in my town when, out of the blue, the hospital discharge planner called me at Noon to say my father was being discharged later that day – in fact, no later than seven p.m.

The hospital informed me unless I picked him by seven – difficult because I lived four hours away – they would transfer him to a local nursing home. When I asked if he could be transferred to the hospital's inpatient rehab unit so he could begin rehab, I was told that, "Medicare (and by extension, my father's top-of-the-line secondary insurance) does not pay for inpatient rehab." This was, and still is, a lie. And yes, there were beds available; that was never an issue. I checked on this through another source. Simply put: The hospital wanted to get rid of him as a patient, and yet would not give me more detailed medical or discharge information.

To this day I still believe the real reason for their lie and the lack of cooperation was that the hospital did not want to bother with an elderly, confused Hispanic man. Unfortunately, these situations do happen in healthcare: Sometimes due to a patient's minority status; sometimes because they are aggressive or difficult to manage; or sometimes because they need expensive medical treatments the facility does not want to get involved with for one reason or another.

Completely under the gun, I finalized arrangements for a skilled nursing facility in my hometown to accept my father late that night. Then, I changed my work schedule and drove the four hours with my husband in the car to pick up my dad.

I found my father sedated, weak, and not able to stand without two people holding him. It was clear he had barely eaten for days, and how he was "ready for discharge" remains a mystery. Thankfully, the nurses, who had not been alerted about his discharge, helped me dress him and get him in a wheelchair.

My husband and I were on our own for when it came to getting my father into my car. We managed, and I drove alone across the state as fast as I could to get him admitted into the rehab facility that night. Every minute on that drive I worried about my dad having a medical emergency. Or, what if he had to do something so seemingly simple as go to the bathroom? I would have to figure out how to get him out of the car all the way to a bathroom and back by myself since my husband stayed behind to drive my father's car the next morning.

Sure, I could have made a stink with the hospital about my father not being ready for discharge. Or, I could have let them transfer him to a nearby nursing home and make arrangements thereafter for a costly and stressful (to my father) transfer. But frankly, I no longer trusted that hospital. I also wanted my father near me right away so I could get a handle on what was happening medically and how best to help him.

As it turned out, my father had lost over thirty pounds because he could not eat, and his labs were in disarray. He had been skipping his cardiac medications because he couldn't remember what to take when, or whether he had already taken them. I also discovered he'd been in two minor car accidents, and made a mess of his finances because he ran out of checks and started using credit card checks that arrived in a promotion because to a demented mind, a check is a check. He even forgot to pay his property taxes, which is evidence of more dementia at work since this was completely out of character for him. I had to quickly get legal control over his healthcare and finances in order to correct this state of affairs.

This is the kind of situation that happens regularly with an elderly parent: They slowly decline, and develop serious medical conditions and possibly dementia. Then they can no longer take care of the basics like finances, food, medications or medical appointments, but will tell no one, much less ask

for help. And if their adult children try to help, they'll rebuff them in one way or another, either out of pride, distrust, or the typical unwillingness to admit age-related decline and helplessness.

Initially, my sick father did not adapt to his nursing home, exhibiting paranoia and agitation. He was unable to remember where he was or what happened, and calmed down only when he saw me. Within a week he was hospitalized again, and was later discharged back into rehab. At that time, he was feeling better, and his labs were more normal. He was calmer with no paranoia or agitation thanks to appropriate medication, more alert, and able to participate fully in rehab.

My dad fell several times during those first couple of months when he tried to go to the bathroom by himself, impatient as always and forgetting his legs no longer worked as they used to. Over time he regained his appetite and weight, and learned to walk again. But due to his advancing dementia and heart condition, he was transferred into long-term care where he was a model resident for over four years until his death.

As for me, I had to apply everything I'd learned during the fifteen years I'd already spent in nursing homes to ensure he was well taken care of and as content and comfortable as possible. Initially, I visited my father daily, varying my times so I knew what was happening throughout the day, night, and on weekends. I spoke to his nurses, aides, and rehab therapists regularly. I tracked his medications, labs, and medical care, and with the competent assistance of a psychiatric nurse practitioner, his psychotropic medications were decreased without any side effects down to one low dose anti-depressant.

With my husband's assistance, we took over my father's financial, insurance, and legal matters. I also made a point of explaining (and repeating) in simple language what was happening and also getting my father's input wherever indicated. I wanted him to feel he was being looked after yet also had a say in his life and over his body. But for the sake of expediency and to lower the stress and avoid needless conflict between me and my independent-minded father, I had to repeatedly choose what to address and what to let slide by prioritizing what was most important. I made these types of choices for the rest of his life; it's the nature of coping with age-related decline and nursing home placement.

In the beginning, handling my father's care and being his advocate was stressful and time-consuming. But as my father transitioned into long-term care, it became easier. In subsequent chapters, I'll return to his journey as a long-term care resident as well as my journey as a care manager so you can learn from us, and perhaps avoid some mistakes and experience a little less heartache.

In sum: If you ever need to be an advocate for the elderly, be mindful of three key areas. First, learn as much as you can about the elder healthcare issues and choices so you will be (somewhat) prepared when the time comes, and it will always be at a moment's notice.

Second, when the crisis erupts, seek as much information as possible regarding their medical status and needs (assuming you have the legal right to medical information and decision-making); prioritize what needs to handled now and what can wait; separate out what you want from what is best for your resident; don't lose sight of the fact there are choices although never as many or as ideal as you would like; and that your loved one does have rights.

Third, take good care of yourself; this will be more stressful, confusing, and challenging than you can imagine. The situation will take time to clarify regarding the direction it's going and what your role will be or can be. Don't wallow in "What ifs," "shoulds," try to assign blame, or figure out the ultimate "Why" that answers every question. Just continue to move forward as best you can in any given moment.

When "Hardcore" Advocacy is Imperative

So far, we've progressed from runaway advocacy where the family member loses sight of the resident's desires, to advocating for a 'younger,' more alert patient, to advocating on behalf of an elderly, incapacitated loved one. Now we'll focus on what I refer to as "hardcore" advocacy, i.e., relentless advocacy on behalf of an "old-old" parent in rehab who cannot speak up for themselves.

A colleague's eighty-nine-year-old mother, Rachel, underwent emergency abdominal surgery and was later transferred to a rehab unit. Unbeknownst to her children, she and her husband had changed their insurance to a Medicare Advantage plan, i.e., a HMO that replaces Medicare and offers lower cost to the participant. This lower cost is often the drawing card that convinces people to sign up (as is as the influence of aggressive HMO salesmen, who promise the world but are not there to deliver services when they are needed the most).

A few days after Rachel's surgery, the HMO told the facility and my friend Bob, who lived out of town from his mother, they were discharging his mother home because "she could walk two hundred feet." What was the reality?

Rachel was bedbound and could not do anything for herself, much less walk two hundred feet. So Bob demanded – yes, *demanded* – his mother be evaluated by rehab in his presence the following day. However, for this to be possible, he had to leave his home and work the next day, and drive several hours to be there for the evaluation. The HMO representative was also present as well as for the evaluation.

As Bob expected, his mother could not walk at all. My colleague demanded an extension of her stay, and basically had to throw a tantrum to get the HMO to extend Rachel's rehab overage for an additional seven days. It was solely due to Bob's extreme but essential efforts – since the nursing home is basically powerless in this situation – that the HMO covered another three weeks, one week at a time, one tantrum at a time. Bob's mother thereafter was able to rehab and return home.

The general rule when you need to employ hardcore advocacy is not to throw tantrums, threaten, yell, or emotionally abuse or put down representatives of HMOs or other third party payers. After all, the employees of such organizations are human beings too, even if they are the face of the insurance carrier. **But sometimes a demanding, angry outburst is all that stands between an "unsafe discharge" that will result in falls, broken bones, and greater health problems, and a chance for the elder to do rehab and resume independent living.**

Health insurance and HMOs are in business to make money, their primary focus on short-term profits. They are not an altruistic charity, and do not care about an individual's welfare or even what is the most effective means to prevent future and costlier healthcare. Rather, the focus of the HMO is on the *immediate* situation and cost savings rather than approving the medically necessary care the resident is legally entitled to have.

Furthermore, the HMO representative is usually following written "medical necessity" standards created solely by the HMO and may know very little about rehab for the elderly or what's needed to optimize the chances of an elder's recovery and successful return home. For example, Medicare Advantage HMOs have denied continued rehab past day seven for stroke victims, even though such residents are barely able to stand, walk, or do the most basic of daily tasks. So while demands, tantrums, and ultimatums are not the best approach in general (and certainly not the most diplomatic), sometimes this is the only approach that will work on behalf of an infirmed, elderly resident who is at the mercy of others.

In sum: If you find yourself the care manager of your parent's hospitalization and rehab, etc., educate yourself as

to the details of their medical coverage and be a strong, outspoken advocate if that is what's needed. If they are denied coverage as in the example above, remember you can file appeals on their behalf as well as contact higher levels in the HMO or insurance carrier, including requesting (or demanding if necessary) a doctor-to-doctor review. Also, you can contact your local Ombudsman (the nursing home will have contact information), or consult a healthcare or elder law attorney.

Denial of Mental Health Evaluations & Services

There's no question psychological services can help correct a resident's mistaken approach to rehab, enhance recovery, and save the Medicare HMO money. This is especially important since the average "length of stay" in rehab is decreasing, which places more pressure on the resident to do rehab right from the very beginning and improve quickly. But Medicare Advantage HMOs view the situation differently despite research data and clinical experience to the contrary. As a result, these HMOs routinely state they do not cover psychological services in a nursing home when they by law they are required to do so.

Over the past twenty years I and other psychologists have chosen to provide what ultimately have amounted to thousands of free services because an HMO refused to pay for mental health services, even if they authorized the services initially. (Be aware that an HMO authorization is no guarantee of actual payment.) In addition, obtaining an authorization is becoming more difficult and time-consuming for the nursing home, and psychologists by themselves cannot request authorization or otherwise intervene.

In one recent case, the HMO refused authorization – yet told the facility social worker to ask the psychologist if they would do the consult for free since they "...sometimes did that." As a result of these actions, I, like a growing number of psychologists, recently curtailed providing free services to HMO residents. Additionally, many physicians have stopped accepting Medicare Advantage HMO patients into their medical practices for similar reasons.

Unfortunately, neither the rehab facility nor the healthcare provider are able to counter these denials or outright refusals to provide or pay services for mental health services. One possible solution is for rehab/skilled nursing homes, as part of their contracts with Medicare HMOs, to negotiate that authorization for psychological services be automatically approved for up to three sessions in order to resolve a crisis and improve rehab participation and success. After all, Medicare HMOs need facilities that can provide effective rehab for their infirmed elderly members just as much as facilities need HMO business. In addition, employers could also negotiate with their HMO that they cover psychological services which actually costs very little; and in a crisis, requiring psychological services in skilled nursing rehab provides great benefit.

People sometimes think healthcare professionals who care should continue to provide free services even if it significantly impacts their income. But would you work five days a week for four day's pay and assume all liability, so a for-profit corporation could make more money? I doubt anyone would answer yes to this question.

At this point, there is basically nothing psychologists can do to remedy the situation because we have no power or leverage against an HMO who refuses to cover mental health services. Consequently, it's in the hands of families, employers, and the general public to advocate for HMO mental health coverage. In the past twenty years, I have never seen or heard of a family member lobby an HMO for authorization and payment for psychological services. And few if any families are in a position to pay for these services out of their own pocket, nor should they when the elderly individual has Medicare coverage that's supposed to cover these services.

> Warriors are not what you think of as warriors. The warrior is not someone who fights, for no one has the right to take another life. The warrior, for us, is the one who sacrifices himself for the good of others. His task is to take care of the elderly, the defenseless, those who cannot provide for themselves, and above all, the children, the future of humanity.
> ~ Sitting Bull

The Thin Veil of Racism

Like every other country, the United States harbors racism and prejudice in one form or another. It's a basic psychological fact that if someone is part of unknown groups and is perceived as threatening in any way, we will reject and treat them as less than fully human. Of course, this depends heavily on our early conditioning and can be more or less prominent as a result. It would be preferable if prejudice didn't exist in healthcare, but prejudice does exist as research and clinical experience has shown. For example, two research studies have found that minorities, especially "Black" men, receive less medical care than "Whites" (who received the highest level of care of any racial or ethnic group).

Not surprisingly, racism will show itself in rehab and nursing homes because they also reflect our nation's history and unresolved issues. In Florida, most aides will be "Black" or "Hispanic," and some do not speak English well despite their State certification and residency status. Residents, however, are primarily "White" and most have lived the majority of their lives outside Florida and its diverse population. In addition, many are of an older generation that did not grow up in close contact with minorities; nor are they tech- and social-media savvy, something that well might widen their world view. This is not to say racism is confined to the elderly because a quick look at the news, U.S. as well as foreign, will prove otherwise.

In nursing homes, the prejudice they harbor will manifest in the residents' behavior and name-calling toward minority staff, especially the aides who provide their daily care. Here are a few examples I've encountered so you can get a sense of what happens.

One male resident ranted and raged against his daytime aide, saying that because of how she walked in the door and her hairstyle that meant she was "low class" and "lazy," and "never did what he wanted." Another man angrily complained about various minority aides, calling them part of "the Haitian clique." This resident went on to make a list of four aides who were acceptable to him, demanding that the facility only schedule those aides to care for him 24/7.

Of course, this type of personalized scheduling is impossible: Many factors go into staff scheduling in a large facility, and catering to one resident is not possible or even desirable since it would confirm for a resident that they can dictate their care. This is not to say a skill nursing home does not make staff changes. But when they are made, it is not to cater to prejudice and/or unreasonable ultimatums.

> Racial prejudice, anti-Semitism, or hatred of anyone
> with different beliefs has no place in the human mind
> or heart.
> ~ Billy Graham

Another rehab resident named Eric showed a different aspect of this issue. He complained about the minority aides, saying that

"...he couldn't understand what they said." Yet he was overlooking his own hearing impairment. In fact, it is quite common that residents seldom recognize their healing loss and its effects on interpersonal communication.

This resident would also rant about all "the illegals" that were taking the CNA (certified nursing assistant or aide) jobs, asking why the nursing home had to hire them. Then he'd go on another rant about "illegals" in general, complaining they were using Medicare money for their rehabs, which "...just wasn't right."

I decided to correct the erroneous information and assumptions Eric had gleaned from the talk shows he often watched and told me about. I told him that in Florida, no "illegal immigrant" can work in a nursing home as facilities run background checks. I informed him that rehab facilities hire more minority aides because "Whites" do not want the jobs. Lastly, no "illegal" can ever receive a Medicare-paid rehab. He was shocked, and so I asked him, "Do you know how Americans qualify for Medicare?"

Like most, this elderly resident did not know the answer even though he'd been a successful businessman with many employees. I briefly explained that an "illegal immigrant" cannot get a Social Security number and as a result does not pay into the Social Security/Medicare system. And if they don't pay in to the system, they get no benefits, like the (expensive) rehab he was receiving. In addition, some "White," native-born U.S. citizens also do not pay into the system for one reason or another, and they also do not receive those benefits. Eric was dumbfounded by this news.

I suggested that whatever he hears on TV talk shows, he should check out and get the facts, and to definitely not let what "talking heads" on TV say for their own income interfere with his recovery and rehab. He got that, and from then on he focused solely on his rehab.

On the other side of the coin, I've talked to elderly gay men who were pleasantly surprised they and their partners did not experience the prejudice they were afraid would occur in a facility. In my experience since the early 1990s, there has been remarkably little prejudice and racism leveled against residents by staff, even toward those residents who are overtly prejudiced and use racial epithets, including the "N-word."

When this name-calling happens, however, I remind staff as well as myself, because I have been on the receiving end of ethnic hostility, that what the resident says reflects the resident, *not them*. If staff takes in or internalizes any insult, their self-esteem is suddenly at stake and that hurts, and stress and anger usually follow which in turn reduces their effectiveness in providing resident care.

I also counsel the name-calling residents, informing them they have the right to think however they please, but if they verbalize racial hate, there will be problems, as well as intervention by the administration. After all, they are living in a facility with many different types of people, and they all need the assistance that is being given to them by the minority staff. Moreover, I tell the residents that their priority and emphasis needs to be on their recovery and rehab, and nothing else. That's the main point, and rehab residents usually get it.

In the event you find your resident leveling racism at staff or other residents, remind your loved one of the need for an attitude that will foster a more effective rehab for themselves. And, that hatred and hostility only begets hostility, not kindness, understanding, and compassionate care.

> Prejudice of any kind implies that you are identified
> with the thinking mind. It means you don't see the
> other human being anymore, but only your own
> concept of that human being. To reduce the aliveness
> of another human being to a concept is already a
> form of violence.
> ~ Eckhart Tolle

"What Would You Do?"

Let's complete our survey of the rehab puzzle with another example. As we go through this example, think about how you might intervene. First, let's learn a little about Charlie, a new nursing home resident admitted after three weeks in inpatient rehab following a stroke.

Charlie was eighty-six, happily married for many years with three children and six grandchildren, all of whom lived out of state. He enjoyed his retirement from the successful business he built "from scratch" with twice-weekly golf and dining out with friends. Unfortunately, Charlie had a "big stroke," ending up with paralysis of his left side, difficulty talking, obvious depression, and frequent tears he could not stop.

When I met Charlie, he had to be lifted out of bed and into a wheel-chair, and still wore diapers although he was beginning to use a urinal. He let me know he "hated" his condition; it "shouldn't have happened;" he "didn't deserve it;" and he wanted to be "the man he used to be," and anything less was "unacceptable."

Charlie told me he wasn't going to "be like the rest of them in the nursing home." He went on to explain that meant infirmed elderly residents who "couldn't do anything and were slumped over in their wheel-chairs, drool coming out of their mouths." Furthermore, he was not going to use a walker to go into a restaurant, adding that was for "suckers" and "poor bastards."

What would you focus on first?

With Charlie there are several avenues to consider, but first I needed ask him a few more questions to get a handle on what might work best. I asked him to tell me little bit more about what happened in order to let him tell his story. Like many, Charlie had no warning a stroke was underway and went to the ER because he felt "funny" all day. Then he said the neurologist in the hospital told him he could recover "90 percent" of his functioning.

Charlie added, "I can accept 90 percent," and tried to produce a smile. Then he said with determination, "I'm going to walk out of here, doc."

We talked about his depression, tears streaming down his face as he spoke of all he "had lost," as, for example, he would never be able to play golf again. Charlie was an active, burly man, and he insisted he'd "never, ever been a crier." He added, "I won't take any depression pills," and made a point to look me in the eye as he said this.

"It's a character thing, like it says you're weak or defective somehow?" I asked.

Charlie nodded. Some elderly residents feel that taking antidepressants reflects a character weakness or flaw. In "their time," people toughed it out and handled life themselves, and didn't rely on help from a bottle of pills. They feel taking antidepressants threatens their sense of themselves, their self-esteem, and that elusive feeling of being in control of their lives.

In rehab, Charlie was doing all right, but his motivation and effort were not what his therapists would have liked. They also reported he often made negative, "giving up" comments and had be coaxed to finish his sessions. Charlie especially didn't like Speech Therapy, telling his therapist every day it was "beneath him," even as he made daily progress he could see.

And Charlie's wife? She was eighty-four, with chronic health problems that were managed. But now she was at wit's end, saying Charlie was "more negative and close-minded" than she'd ever seen him. She implored me to help him because he wasn't listening to her or anyone else. Regrettably, the stress of Charlie's stroke and his attitude took a toll other her health and she ended up in the hospital for a few days – something that's happened to other spouses in similar situations.

If Charlie was your spouse, partner or parent, what would you say to him?

With Charlie, there were two main issues that immediately stood out: depression and crying episodes which are unusual for a man (although less so after a stroke in certain areas of the brain), and indifferent rehab participation.

With a stroke, rehab is long and slow, and always much slower than the resident expects. In addition, almost all stroke patients experience depression to one degree or another, and for some it can be lifelong if they have to live with significant disability and a negative change in their lifestyle, activities, and sense of themselves. It looked as if Charlie was heading into this latter group, especially since he would not consider anti-depressants and could not control his crying. *But where and how should we start to change the path Charlie was on?*

First: *With a man like Charlie, it's prudent to avoid confronting his pride and inflexibility head on, especially when it's already threatened by the stroke.*

Second: *When and what to say to help can sometimes be revealed by what the resident repeats with emotion.* In Charlie's case, he'd already stated several different issues or opinions where we could intervene, but I had to choose one or two and see how he responded. So I asked him about a couple of items that reflected his inflexible and unrealistic expectations, knowing they were impacting his rehab participation. I focused on his expectations since they are often the key that opens the door to a new attitude. I decided to ask Charlie about what the neurologist had told him since that had made such an impression.

"Charlie, the neurologist in the hospital said you could recover to 90 percent. What if it's 85 percent, could you live with that?"

"Hmm, yes, 85 percent is OK." Charlie wrinkled his brow, baffled by the question.

"How about 80 percent. Could you live with that?"

"Oh, no, no," Charlie said quickly, shaking his head. "No. No."

We obviously had gone past his comfort zone, and now I knew I had to take it slow and easy with Charlie. Yet we had opened the door a little to another possibility (85 percent). In so doing, I could then address how to do rehab right and hopefully get to the magical 90 percent and avoid the 80 percent he felt was unacceptable. Having unearthed this information, I now could give Charlie concrete "jobs" or tasks to do every day.

It's important to remember that with elderly rehab residents who still feel unwell and frightened by what is happening to them, and whose brain is not functioning anywhere near its best, less is often more. Focus on the basics over and over again, and in simple language so the impaired mind can take in the information.

I also decided to explore another rigid opinion or expectation Charlie repeated several times – namely, that he was never going into a restaurant with a walker because that was for "poor bastards."

I began by telling him a little of my father's journey in rehab to give him hope that like my father, he could recover his walking ability with hard work in therapy.

Charlie liked that, nodding and trying to smile despite his stroke impairment. Then I went one step further, and told him that in the four and a half years my father was in long-term care we regularly went to lunch at his favorite restaurant and he walked in with his walker.

"So what's this about people with walkers being "poor bastards"? My father loved going out to eat, and never had a problem with his walker in public."

Charlie shook his head emphatically, and said, "Let's forget about your father."

Once again, we had gone past Charlie's comfort zone by presenting new information that went against an old, inflexible opinion. Here, I followed Charlie's lead and moved on to his next topic, but I had done enough. Charlie now had another perspective based on someone else's experience who had gone before him, and this showed him not only the way out of his predicament, but that it could be done.

WHAT WOULD YOU DO?

The sky isn't the limit: the mind that sees the sky is the limit.
~ Byron Katie

Since Charlie continued to cry daily over the next few weeks, the issue of an anti-depressant hovered. Men of his generation seldom cry like Charlie did, and even though it was related to his stroke, the fact his mood was noticeably depressed and could well affect his recovery made it an issue that couldn't be dismissed. Crying in a man his age under these circumstances usually calls for medication because the depression is apt to worsen and interfere with recovery if not resolved quickly.

Anti-depressants given to a stroke patient early on actually helps them heal faster. And like the vast majority of his generation, Charlie was not interested, capable, or practiced in using more sophisticated psychological/cognitive techniques to address his depression.

Charlie's wife and his nurses also thought he should take anti-depressants. But Charlie was adamant he wouldn't take "any depression pills" for any reason, including the stroke, still thinking his character was at stake. His attending physician couldn't prescribe anti-depressants because Charlie tracked his medications carefully and he also had the right to refuse medications.

What more could we do to help Charlie? Here are some options. Which one would you choose?

1. Get his wife and three adult children to make a united campaign to convince Charlie that taking anti-depressants would be helpful and he needs to agree.

2. Ask the attending physician to prescribe an anti-depressant that would also aid his sleep problems and not mention that it's primarily for depression.

3. Let Charlie be. Since he's entitled to refuse medications, let him flounder in his depression because he'll only make

a difficult problem worse with repeated refusals and arguments.

4. Don't bother with the issue since Charlie was projected to go home in two months and any confrontation would likely make him 'dig in his heels' and work against his rehab.

5. Keep chipping away at his negative opinions and expectations in the hope that will curb his depression and crying jags.

6. Explain again (and again) why an anti-depressant would benefit him in the hope he would finally see the light. Educate him that this crying was caused by the stroke as well as his reactions to it and his rehab confinement. In other words, emphasize the physical cause to offset the possibility Charlie would see this information as emasculating or criticizing his character.

7. Tell Charlie to "suck it up" and be the strong man he thinks he is and "stop bothering his wife with all his complaints and negative thinking. It's not her job to make him feel better, even though that's what she's always done." (I've heard some version of this from many adult children frustrated with their parent's reaction.)

8. Come up with a new idea no one has ever thought of before, and quickly.

What I focused on was a combination of number 5, 6, and 7. I explained to Charlie that if he did not agree to an anti-depressant, and that was his right and it would be respected, he would need to basically manage his depression and crying through his own inner strength. I also urged Charlie to take his time and think about the pros and cons of taking an anti-depressant and to not dismiss it out of hand. And, that whatever he decided, he could always change his mind in the future.

In this case, Charlie decided against an anti-depressant, so I reminded him that doing so meant he would need to actively help himself – and that might mean he needed to "tough it out" and "not give in" to the crying and his negative, pessimistic thinking. I said it in this language *only because it matched Charlie's own word choices* even though it is not a word choice I recommend or normally use.

So what happened to Charlie? He stopped crying except when he thought of his children who flew into town as a birthday surprise. During this visit, he spent hours talking with his children, and felt closer than ever before. He later went to his favorite burger joint with his son using his walker outside the facility for the first time. Charlie's rehab took off, and after another month, he went home walking with a cane.

By then Charlie was able to do all his ADLs (activities of daily living, such as using the bathroom, dressing, showering, etc.). Although Charlie did not reach the 90 percent mark he coveted and he was still a bit unsteady, he came close to his goal and was pleased.

Moreover, Charlie opened his heart with gratitude for every small measure of progress and for his second chance at life. He still cried a little, but no longer thought his tears were unmanly because now they were tears of love and appreciation for his wife and family.

> There's nothing that cleanses your soul like getting the hell kicked out of you.
> ~ Woody Hayes

Time-Tested Tips

- If you're the care manager for your loved one, be aware your role will be different for a younger, more alert rehab resident as opposed to an elderly resident. Educate yourself, though, as to each role and approach so you can make more informed decisions in order to better help your loved one.

- Be aware of the limits of advocacy, and spend some time learning how to be a more effective, perhaps even a subtle advocate. You can only do what you can do, not necessarily what you *think* you should do or want to do. You will not be able to fix everything, or make your loved one's rehab and recovery perfect, or save them from all their pain and suffering.

If they complain about the staff or the facility, and chances are they will, *get the facts before jumping to conclusions or letting your anger or fear rule the day*. Your loved one may be right and something needs to be changed, *but they could be wrong because their memory is impaired by their illness, anesthesia and other drugs, or they are victims of their prejudices or own unrealistic expectations.*

For example, I once entered a resident's room and she immediately began complaining that the staff *always* took "over an hour" to answer her call light. She needed them right now, she repeated, but once again, they hadn't responded. However, I noticed she hadn't pressed the call light, so I pressed it and noted the time. When the aide came in, the resident said, "See, it was an hour!"

I answered, "No, it was seven minutes. I timed it."

The lesson here is *when we're sick and waiting on someone else to help us, it feels as if every minute is an hour, every hour is a day, every day is a week, and so on. In light of that, don't believe everything you hear, but do check it out and get the facts.*

- Please remember to ask the resident what they want in terms of medical treatments, etc. It's their body and their life, so what do they want? Is what they want feasible and without serious side effects or repercussions? Are there other options? Can your elderly resident understand the issues involved as well as the pros and cons of every treatment choice?

- If they are unable to voice their preferences and choices, and you have the legal right to do so in their name, consider what they've said in the past as well as any answers to the questions above. Discuss the pros and cons of every choice with their physician, and ask for specifics if you're unclear what each choice involves.

- Avoid being a nag or a Drill Sergeant. That never works, and it will stress you out and cause needless friction with your loved one.

- **4 - 4 Breathing:** Breathe in slowly and gently to a count of 4.

    Imagine your breath going all the way down to your belly button.

Then purse your lips and exhale slowly and gently for a count of 4,
imagining your breath flowing outward like a soft breeze,
leaving in its wake an alert mind and a relaxed, alive body.

>Every breath we take, every step we take can be filled
>with peace, joy and serenity.
>~ Thich Nhat Hanh

Chapter 6
Making and Accepting Hard Choices

"There's a lot of love here," Sam said, waving his brush around, drops of paint falling onto his well-worn, paint splattered tee shirt.

I had met Sam, the lone painter contracted to repaint the interior of a large nursing home, a month earlier. On his first day on the job he'd told me, "I've never been inside a nursing home. I've never seen this many old, sick people before."

Like most people, Sam had only heard horror stories about "smelly" nursing homes and abusive and unconcerned staff. He personally had never known or helped care for an elderly, infirmed individual.

"I don't know how y'all do it," he added, and shook his head. "I can't wait to finish this job and go back to painting houses. No sick people there."

Everyday Sam came to work at eight sharp and meticulously laid out his tarp, paints, and brushes. He started with the third floor and slowly worked his way down, trying to focus only on his job, but the world around him enveloped him nonetheless. Every week we spoke as we both went about our business; and I tried to encourage him and fend off his fear.

"You're comfortable here now," I observed. "What made the difference for you?"

"The more time I spent here and saw what y'all are doing, and got to know some of the residents and the people who work here, the more I could see the love that was going around. Sure they're old and sick and can't do much anymore, sure the staff is too busy, but there's love here...real love." Sam shared a toothy smile. "I'm going to miss this place."

Sam said it best: There is a lot of love in a nursing home that can't be seen at first blush when the vast ocean of human frailty seems ready to engulf us, and we can't imagine there ever being any joy or laughter within such walls. But if you're lucky and do spend some time in a nursing home and get to know some of the staff and residents, you'll begin to see love in one of its many disguises – just like Sam learned to do.

> Kindness in words creates confidence.
> Kindness in thinking creates profoundness.
> Kindness in giving creates love.
> ~ Lao Tzu

Kindness When You Least Expect It

At the start of her stay, one elderly rehab resident recovering from ankle surgery said she "tried not to look at" the sicker long-term residents because they made her so sad. She stayed in her room with the door closed as much as possible, venturing out only for her rehab. By the end of her stay, her outlook had changed, and her initial depression and isolated time spent in her room were things of the past.

"Early one morning, I was roaming the halls because I couldn't sleep, wishing for my morning cup of coffee and toast. I hadn't had any for a month," she began. "One of the young black fellas from the kitchen saw me and came out to see if I needed anything. I said "No," and told him how much I missed my morning toast with butter and jam. He said to go wait in the dining room, and went back to the kitchen. A few minutes later he came back with fresh coffee, buttered toast and strawberry jam. He didn't have to do that. It wasn't his job, but he did it anyway." She smiled, her soft brown eyes twinkling.

"That kindness made my day, and there's a lot of that here. I thought my life was over when I broke my ankle and couldn't even go to the bathroom by myself, much less wipe myself, but now I see there's more living left to do. Maybe I can pass along a little kindness that will brightened someone's day. I always thought helping someone had to be big, but now I see that it can be very small," she added.

As my rehab friend found out, kindness comes in all sorts of packages, mostly small and unadorned. But in the midst of our busy lives we tend to overlook kindness, even discard it as trivial and unimportant. Sometimes if we're lucky, we can be surprised and graced by its simple presence in a nursing home.

As Friar Richard Rohr reminds us, "Self-worth is not created; it is discovered." To that we might add, love is not created, it is rediscovered, nurtured, and then shared.

Finding love and kindness in a nursing home is not something a new rehab or long-term care resident or their family sees or are looking for. What sends people into long-term care is illness severe enough that daily living without a significant amount of assistance is impossible or unsafe. Often elderly spouses and other family members have to admit they can no longer provide the care and supervision that's needed. This may also mean they have to finally accept the reality of a diagnosis such as advanced Alzheimer's disease, Parkinson's, or ALS that they've tried hard to dismiss…until one day it could no longer be denied.

It's always a sad and sobering day when it becomes clear a decision must be made and the only viable choice is long-term care in a nursing home. On that day we come face to face with not only our loved one's mortality, but also our own.

Responding to "Why Can't I Go Home?"

This is probably the hardest question a family member has to face. Sometimes it's a question that is repeated over and over by a resident who will not or cannot accept the answer because it's not what they desire or can see for themselves.

How do you answer the question "Why can't I go home?" if the rehab resident continues to deny their decline and infirmity?

How do you tell them they can't be trusted to live alone because they can't remember enough to turn off the stove or pay their bills, much less drive safely or manage their medications, and you live across the country and can't help?

How do you tell them they've permanently lost their independence, as well as the home they've lived in for years? Or that they won't be recovering enough to go home, despite their hard work in rehab and the marvels of modern medicine.

How do you tell your spouse of half a century that you can't take care of him anymore as you promised on your wedding day?

How do you tell your mother who expects you to take care of her until her death…like she took care of grandma?

How do you tell your elderly once-alcoholic father who is berating you like he used to that he'll have to make the facility his new home and live by the rules of others?

How do you tell any of them that they have to live in an institution for the rest of their lives? How do you tell them when they, as well as you, think life dealt them a bad hand they didn't deserve?

For most residents, transfer into long-term care from an unsuccessful or partially successful rehab is for the rest of their lives. Only a small percentage can later go home to live on their own, or with some help. By and large, residents know this even if they have some dementia and can't remember today's date, the names of their grandchildren, or their medical condition. Every resident also seems to harbor the belief that living in a nursing home is, "…the worst fate possible" and something they never dreamed would happen to them. Yet now it has, and they're powerless to change this fate.

Sometimes, a long-term care resident will come into a facility directly from home, and it's always because of a serious health decline and safety concerns. Most recognize that the nursing home will be their home until the day they die; and on some level they know this even if they are not conscious of this reality.

Other residents simply cannot accept long-term care forever, so they deny their reality, weaving a fantasy that's improbable but gets them though the day. For example, one woman with a severe stroke who needed total care said, "I have to have a goal: to go home, back to my life. Or else, I can't take living here."

And until her death seven years later she held on to that goal, a goal both her family and staff knew was impossible.

What should have the family or staff told her the day she transferred to long-term care? What should they have said throughout those seven long years when she repeatedly said she wanted to go home?

Since the transfer into long-term care covers a large variety of residents and situations, there is no one set way to manage and handle this situation. So below I'll discuss common issues and ways to handle them.

As to the woman with the stroke who said she would "never accept" long-term placement, I recommended that everyone respect what she needed, and that was her dream to go home, however elusive and impractical. Whenever she brought it up, I and the rest of the staff would listen until she moved on to other areas of her current life. She knew what had to happen before she could leave the nursing home, so there was no point to repeating the obvious, except to puncture her dream and hurt her. She had more than enough to contend with, already having lost her health, independence, home, and small hair salon in the blink of an eye.

> Do not dwell in the past, do not dream of the future,
> concentrate the mind on the present moment.
> ~ Buddha

Waiting to Tell

As mentioned previously, I do not recommend telling a rehab resident they are going to stay in the nursing home long-term until they are *almost finished with their rehab*. The reason is that many will throttle back their rehab efforts as they react to the unexpected news and have to adjust their expectations.

Some can accept the news of long-term care with grace and understanding, but others will get depressed and give up. Some will become angry, belligerent, and uncooperative – none of this will serve them since the goal of rehab (regardless of where they end up) is to get the resident as strong and as mobile as possible. Becoming stronger and more mobile will assist them in their daily activities, as well as lessen pain and stiffness, decrease the possibility of pressure sores, and increase their sense of satisfaction and peace.

For rehab residents who end up in long-term care, many will see concrete proof throughout their rehab therapy of what they can and cannot do, and often they start comparing themselves to other residents who make more progress and go home. Little by little, and without their conscious awareness, they are receiving information as to whether or not they can do basic life activities such as get out of bed, walk, do daily toileting, dress, manage medications, and so on. Consequently, some residents already know they cannot go home even before they are told.

This is the easiest situation to manage, because the resident has already made the initial adjustment to long-term care and feels somewhat comfortable with the facility and their care team. In addition, some of these residents feel as if a weight has been taken off when they learn they are going to live in the nursing home. They no longer feel yoked by having to try to do things they no longer can do. They also feel a burden has been taken off their adult children, and this is a relief to them.

Many residents, especially the women, say they do not want to "burden" their children with their care in their old age, desiring them to have lives free from the sacrifice of long-term care giving. Some of these women already know firsthand how much time and energy caregiving consumes, and how much of their own needs and dreams were once brushed aside for the sake of the safety and wellbeing of a loved one.

For other residents, especially those who hold fast to the belief that they will return home, there are two choices: 1) tell them it's a permanent placement, or 2) tell them that it's a temporary one, leaving the door open to the possibility they can return home.

When The Dream Ends

While residents may dream of leaving long-term care, the actual realization of this dream proves slim. Going home is rarely possible, even if sometimes, due to the structured, supportive environment of a nursing home as well as the ongoing medical oversight, the resident actually improves over a period of twelve months or so. They may feel better and become more functional and active, and with that improvement the resident begins thinking they can go home and resume independent living, even if they no longer have a home. What the resident (and sometimes their family) does not realize is how little they do while living in the nursing home, and how supportive and helpful the environment actually is. Thus the resident (and their family) will revisit (sometimes frequently) the question as to why they can't go home, and why they need to live in long-term care.

Let's figure out how to manage this heartbreaking issue through the lens of an actual example that takes into account the perspective of both the infirmed and the caregiver(s).

Marie, age eighty-six, came into rehab after another fall and pneumonia, which required a lengthy rehab. For the last five years,

Marie had been living in Florida with Lucy, her sixty-six-year-old divorced daughter, as she could no longer live alone in her home in Brooklyn, New York. Marie did well enough in her rehab, but could only regain limited standing ability and had to rely on a wheel-chair. In addition, her recent history of falls and generalized weakness signaled that she would have to depend on her daughter Lucy more and more.

Marie fully expected her daughter, now retired from teaching school, to continue taking care of her until her death. As she often said, "I did it for my mother and my husband, and he was no picnic, and she (daughter Lucy) is supposed to do it for me. I'm not going into a nursing home. Maybe I'll go back to Brooklyn, to my old apartment."

So how did Marie's daughter Lucy feel about these things?

According to Lucy, Marie was often "demanding and never satisfied." (This was a lifelong pattern of hers the whole family acknowledged.) Lucy had had enough – but she was a caretaker and a pleaser by nature. If she followed her own desires, Lucy would have to go against her mother's wishes, as well as family and their religious tradition.

So as Marie's discharge date approached, Lucy's guilt and stress grew stronger. All Marie talked about was "going home," oblivious to her own limited physical abilities or Lucy's stress. Lucy wanted her mother to be "understanding and cooperative," as Lucy had knee, shoulder and back problems, and would probably be getting a knee replacement in the future.

Where do we begin? With Marie or Lucy? What issue do we tackle first?

Actually, the most effective place to start is with Lucy. As you read above, Marie didn't think a problem even existed since she believed she was going back home to be taken care of by her daughter. Moreover, Marie was also exhibiting cognitive and memory decline that could be seen in her unrealistic statement that she might go back to her "old Brooklyn apartment" after she had been living with her daughter in another state for the past few years. Think what it would take for anyone to move to another state over a thousand miles away and find an apartment in a state they have not lived in for years? Plus, since all her family lived outside of New York, Marie would have to be able to take complete care of herself and her health (impossible given her infirmity and need for a wheel-chair), find and manage a new apartment, including paying rent and utilities, cooking for herself, and buying furniture, get a set of new doctors, and figure out how to get groceries and prescriptions without a car and a daughter by her side to help.

If you were to ask Marie about the responsibilities the move would entail, she would probably look at you blankly or dismiss the issue. Or else she might say her daughter or other family member would take care of it, or that she took care of herself and the apartment for years, so what's the problem? This is the typical response: Only a few residents are able to recognize they cannot do any of it anymore. But others will make light of any questioning because if they don't, they will have to acknowledge the extent of their decline. And for some, merely suggesting the possibility can also be a way to guilt the family member into saying something like: "Ma, you can't go back to Brooklyn by yourself! You're living with me here!"

Marie is using guilt, along with her unyielding expectation of a *quid pro quo* ("I did, so I get back"), with no thoughts as to whether Lucy had agreed to this or can do it indefinitely, or even any consideration of Lucy's health. This also points to cognitive decline since the person with mild cognitive impairment or dementia does not recognize their own rigid thinking or empathize with the needs and afflictions of others. In short, Marie's thinking style seems to be along the lines of: 'It is because I think and say it is, and it's always been this way, and you owe me.'

As for Lucy, she could use counseling since she has several

issues to address, and these will be a challenge since she still strives to be a "good girl" who pleases her mother and does her duty, while always feeling the tug of guilt. So, where and how should this potential caregiver start making this important decision?

> No one has the power to hurt you. It is only your own
> thinking about someone's actions that can hurt you.
> ~ Epictetus

How to Make a Viable, Conscious Decision

Step One: Consider All Facets.

Lucy, or any family member in this position, needs to be clear regarding the health and functional ability of their loved one, as well as themselves if they are the potential caregiver option.

Below is a list of basic questions they – or you – should have the answers to in order to go on to the next steps of managing the guilt that invariably comes with making the decision.

1. *What can the resident do?*

If you or another family can't answer that in detail about the resident or you are unsure, a good source of information is the rehab and nursing staff. They can voice their assessments and experience with the resident to you. For example, if they respond that the resident is "total care," that's exactly what it means: The resident cannot do much of anything by themselves. So if they are going home, the family (or full-time healthcare aides) must be able to provide that level of daily care for them.

If family is still unclear after receiving the staff's report, stay and observe what the aide does to get a resident ready in the morning to go to rehab, including toileting and food management. To further get a complete and total picture of the support the resident needs, move on to #2.

2. *What kind of help does the resident need? Can the resident, stand, pivot, and transfer themselves to a wheelchair? Do they use a walker? How well can they walk? Can they transfer themselves to and from the commode? Do they need help wiping themselves clean? Do they use diapers, pull-ups, or other incontinent products? Can they shower, shampoo, or shave themselves? What other kinds of help do they need?*

Make a list of daily living abilities and tasks such as these, and be specific, detailing not only the needs of the resident but actual considerations of whether the family caregiver can do these tasks.

For example, an answer like "Help with getting dressed" would not be specific enough because it does not specify the many steps involved. As a result, it's often helpful to watch how an aide dresses your resident, or think back what it took to dress young children, or what you do in the morning to get ready for work. We do many more steps than any of us realize because they have become second-nature.

"Help dressing" also does not answer whether the caregiver can provide that kind of support presently and maybe indefinitely. For example, a caregiver who cannot bend down or kneel down, or has a bad back, cannot pick up someone's legs to put on shoes, socks or compression stockings, underwear and pants, much less change diapers or pull-ups. If, like Marie above, the resident cannot stand except minimally, and needs help getting in and out of bed, help transferring into and out of a wheelchair as well as down and up from a commode, then the caregiver must be strong enough to do it for the resident. Marie already needs a lot of help, and Lucy's back, shoulder, and knee problems, probably have been aggravated, if not caused, by the strain of helping Marie for the past five years. Also, Lucy at age sixty-six is not the same woman she was five years ago.

Also, observe also whether the resident is overweight or obese. If they cannot help at all and are "dead weight," their body will feel much heavier than it is. Their care will be even harder for a single caregiver to provide and manage.

3. *What does the resident need medically?*

For example, with a diabetic resident, does their sugar need to be checked, and if so, how many times a day? Do they get insulin injections? Again, be specific. Then ask yourself if you, if you are going to be their potential caregiver, can you do this for them day in and day out. Write down your honest feedback.

4. *What do I, the potential home caregiver, need for myself, and how will I get the patient looked after if I am not available?*

Have you thought about what you are going to do during the times when you cannot provide the patient's necessary care due to your own illness, injury, or healthcare appointments; vacation or need for R & R (rest & recuperation); car trouble; job commitments if you're still working, and so on? What support system do you have, if any, for each of these events?

5. *How much supervision will the resident need at home?*

Some residents, such as those with more advanced dementia or stroke-related impairments, cannot be left alone. At all. *Who will supervise them 24/7? Are there other family members or neighbors able to help? Can you count on them long-term? Or, can you afford to hire help?*

6. *What is the resident's basic personality and how are they reacting to their decline? What kind of a patient are they? How do they respond emotionally to illness and pain?*

Some people are cooperative and patient, but others get irritable, impatient, critical, demanding, anxious, whiny, self-pitying, and so on. How would you, as their caregiver, manage, given their temperament and the fact that both of you are stressed?

Marie fell into this latter category of being difficult to care for and live with. So Lucy needs to ask herself whether she can handle that day in and day out without becoming mean and resentful herself.

What's needed most here is a thorough, objective assessment of what the resident needs, as well as an honest assessment of what you can and cannot do, and whether you can live with sacrificing or postponing your own life. Please know there is no shame to be found here if you are not up to the challenge or otherwise incapable of providing the necessary care.

7. *Given your detailed answers, can you as a caregiver provide what the resident needs on a daily basis?*

Consider that the help you provide may mean you are "on" 24 hours a day, 7 days a week, for what maybe years and years. This may mean you, and you alone, must carry the caregiving burden if there is no one else able and ready to help you or you cannot afford to hire help. The question is not whether you would *like* to provide the care, or what you *should* be able to do. Or, what would be best for the resident in an ideal situation, or what your loved one prefers. It is simply *whether you can do it physically, emotionally, and financially, minute by minute, day after day.*

It's a Yes or No question; not an issue of love, caring, or morality.

For Lucy, her answer was "No." In addition, she wanted to be able to do a few things for herself now that she was retired. She felt she had sacrificed herself raising her children and coping with a difficult twenty-year marriage while working full time. Her three children who lived out-of-state were urging her to come visit and spend time with her grandchildren, something Lucy had postponed for years in order to care for Marie. Lucy felt she had done enough and had nothing left to give.

Lucy was able to reach a basic truth about her situation that would guide her decision-making. No, she could not physically and emotionally do Marie's daily caretaking. Yes, she wanted to visit her kids and their families before she got a knee replacement or had other health problems. With these insightful, conscious decisions, Lucy was finally in a position where she could effectively confront her guilt.

> It seems to me that everyone on this planet whom I know or have worked with is suffering from self-hatred and guilt to one degree or another. The more self-hatred and guilt we have, the less our lives work. The less self-hatred and guilt we have, the better our lives work, on all levels.
> ~ Louise L. Hay

Step Two: Manage the Guilt.

Guilt is an emotion that has different facets.

One facet is the "righteous guilt" we may feel over having done something that hurts someone or goes against our moral principles. When this happens we can either make a genuine apology; or make amends to the person we've hurt; or take steps to change our behavior so it's in line with our principles. Hopefully, we learn from our mistake and take that knowledge and awareness into the future so we avoid hurting that person again or others. In this way, guilt serves a useful function by spurring us to more considerate and life-affirming behavior.

Then there is the guilt we feel when we are not living up to an expectation that was placed on us by others early in our lives and we continue to hold over ourselves. This guilt, with all its attendant self-criticisms, is the result of unquestioned beliefs regarding what we should and should not do in order to please and win the love and approval of others, especially our parents. This guilt can be coupled with shame, that deep sense of unworthiness or self-hatred that we're not good enough in some undefined and essential way.

The remedy we most often reach for is to redouble our efforts to satisfy those "shoulds" and expectations. While this may work for a while, it will never be enough no matter how hard or how long we try *because the underlying cause* – an emotional complex that is independent of external reality – *has not been addressed*.

Marie, for example, had a clear expectation that in her family, daughters take care of their parents – and if not, then they're selfish, bad wives and bad daughters. There was no room in Marie's world to take into account individual circumstances, capabilities, health, aging, or personal preferences, much less consider other options.

As for Lucy, her children were repeatedly telling Lucy, "Mom, do something *for yourself*. Come visit us and enjoy yourself finally!" Even Lucy's older brother told her she'd done more than enough for their difficult mother. So Lucy had to choose whether to follow her early programming to avoid her mother's disapproval and pacify her own guilt – or make a conscious choice to respect her own limits and honor what she deeply felt was in her best interest and the interest of her children and grandchildren.

Lucy chose the latter. But it's important to recognize that making a choice does not get rid of the guilt for all time. The guilt can reassert itself, and if it does, do as Lucy did, using these techniques and realizations.

First: Whenever her guilt arose in the future, Lucy reminded herself *to breathe several times, then reaffirm her choice and why she chose it*.

Second: Lucy recognized she had to accept she would probably receive some backlash from her mother. Lucy allowed her mother to have her own emotional reaction, *understanding that even if it was negative, that did not mean she had to "give in" to her mother*.

Third: Lucy accepted the fact that she should not try to change, reason or manipulate Marie into what Lucy wanted, i.e., an "understanding and cooperative" mother. To truly reach some place of harmony between the two of them, she would have to become more conscious and responsible for her choices and expectations, as well as allow Marie to have her emotional reaction without trying to change it.

Viewing the situation from a broader, more universal perspective, you may be wondering what part you should actually play in your resident's reaction to your news that you are unable to become their daily caregiver. Basically nothing, except to give the resident the space and time to experience and express their reaction. That may mean leaving the person alone so they can do that. However, if the patient becomes became enraged or aggressive, then other steps are needed. This includes setting clear limits and leaving as soon as possible since this contains their reaction and helps the resident maintain some control over themselves.

Should you explain to your resident all the reasons why you made the choice you did?

Not particularly, or probably not more than once or a few times if the resident has memory issues. Why? If you were to explain yourself then you would be giving the message that the choice is negotiable. This inevitably leads to the usual back and forth discussion of this choice, as well as never-ending arguments while the resident tries to change a decision they do not like or approve of.

Thus, the question becomes: *Once it is made, is your choice negotiable?*

For many it is not. And in time – sometimes rather quickly – the residents can come to accept the choice. This proved the case with Marie. Why? Because Lucy was clear and unwavering in her conscious choice, and it was not made out of malice, payback, or revenge against Marie.

This does not mean Marie would come to like or approve Lucy's decision. That may never come to pass, but Marie would accept Lucy's choice because they would be no other option. This then opens the door for Marie to begin to make peace with long-term care.

If you follow this straightforward process consistently, you dis-identify from your own programming and "shoulds," and consciously move forward. Every time you do the process, you grow stronger in your own truth, while the "I-should-please" and

"I-feel-so-guilty" pattern grows weaker.

Over time, the guilt and all its accompanying "shoulds" fade into echoes and may even disappear altogether. It's important to dis-empower this guilt pattern so when our long-term care resident dies, we can be at peace without the berating sting of old guilt and "shoulds." And for Marie, this also frees her to move forward and accept her new reality rather than wasting precious time and wasting energy debating whether or not she can go home or trying to manipulate her daughter into taking her in.

To recap succinctly, here's what you should do if you feel guilty about your caregiving choice:

1. *Breathe.* Do the 4 - 4 Breathing technique to relax your mind-body and open yourself to a new possibility. Do it as often as you need to and whenever you feel an emotional charge arise.

2. *State your choice to yourself.* This assumes you have clearly outlined the available choices like we did above with Lucy. If you haven't, go back and do this essential step so you can make a clear, conscious choice.

3. *Remind yourself of the reason(s) why you made that choice.*

4. *Repeat these steps as often as necessary, and always when the guilt pattern emerges.*

> Guilt can prevent us from setting the boundaries that would be in our best interests, and in other people's best interests.
> ~ Melody Beattie

Step Three: Determine the *best* living option for your loved one, given the circumstances AND your caregiving choice.

Lucy thought long and hard about Marie's health, and finally acknowledged that meant long-term care in a nursing home. For someone else, it could be an Assisted Living Facility if they can meet the health and functioning criteria, as well as have the capacity to afford this option.

Step Four: Inform the patient in simple, clear language about the living option decision you have made for them.

Lucy had to tell Marie she was going into a nursing home for the rest of her life. Once again, Lucy had to first be clear about her choice and her reasons for it, and that it was non-negotiable. Lucy then told her mother the discharge plan into long-term care in plain, concrete language that did not blame or berate Marie.

And Marie's response? She was muted in her response, with no hysterics or angry outbursts like Lucy feared, and accepted the discharge plan quickly. This was probably because Marie already knew the reality of her own health, and also sensed the inner strength of Lucy's conscious choice.

What if Marie or any other resident is unaccepting, angry, and argumentative of the care choice that is made?

The response must be to *let the resident have their reaction* – which also means you no longer have to be present. This means: If someone is angry, the general rule is to *let them have their space to be angry*. The resident's anger will decrease and eventually exhaust itself if others do not try to change or overpower them, which results in more conflict and more emotion. If you are with an angry and unaccepting resident, leave politely and let them have their emotions as well as time to mull over the news and their situation.

This is what I did when I told my father he would be staying in long-term care, something he did not want. I told him that because of his medical condition (and I named the primary ones), he would not be able to return to his condo nor could he live with me. I could not provide the care he needed, but I would help him every step of the way. He would not be alone, and I was sorry things didn't work out the way he would have liked. My father made some angry remark I didn't respond to, and then he went quiet. I added that this was difficult news to hear and he probably needed time alone, and I said goodbye. He accepted the news in short order and he was able to make the nursing home his home. And yes, I rehearsed what I wanted to say before I spoke to him, something I recommend family members also do.

> The clearer we get about ourselves,
> the kinder we become.
> ~ Byron Katie

If Indecision, Mixed Messages, and False Hope Rule the Day

What makes this type of care decision more difficult is when the family member vacillates back and forth. In essence saying, "Yes, you have to be in long-term care. No, you don't; you can come home. Yes, I'll take care of you, but oh, I really can't. No, you can't come home. Yes, we'll talk about when you can come home,"' and on and on. There is no clarity or direction here, and the resident is being given false hope.

It's the caregiver's indecision, vacillation and confusion – which are fueled by guilt and "shoulds" – that opens the door to circular arguments and hard feelings. As if that isn't enough, we also expect the resident to be understanding and considerate of us, as well as accept their long-term nursing home placement without giving us any problems. Typically, family members also expect their loved one to be "happy" to live in a nursing home, but this is unrealistic. **We need to give up our expectations as much as they need to give theirs up – perhaps more so.**

I've seen this scenario of mixed messages, indecision, and unrealistic expectations over and over again, and it does not work for anyone.

The process I outlined above does work. Not all the time of

course, or as neatly as it did for Lucy, and not with every resident. But it works because it resolves the basic problem of mixed messages, guilt, and manipulation. After these initial steps are settled, the issue becomes how to make the resident's new home as positive as possible.

Positive Placements

As a general rule, it takes residents several months to adjust to their placement, and this also applies to Assisted Living. A small percentage make the adjustment fairly quickly while some take longer, and some never do. If they do not, that is their choice.

What if the nursing home is only a *temporary* placement? This sometimes happens when the discharge plan is for the resident to return home once certain medical conditions are resolved, or when the spouse or family settles some issue first. In this instance, I suggest the resident be told what the plan is, in simple, concrete language, and what needs to happen or change before they can leave the facility. Over-explaining is more troublesome than focusing on the basics and then allowing the resident to ask questions. It's helpful to leave the discharge date open-ended unless a clear date has already been determined.

If a resident is to transfer out of state to a retirement community or another facility, and there is a holdup with transportation, availability, or some other issue, *give the resident regular updates.* This keeps their spirits up until the transfer happens. In this situation, the majority of residents seem to handle delays fairly well as long as there is not a great deal of anxiety and mixed messages from the family regarding the transfer or delays. As with rehab, focus on the essentials and living in the moment, or doing what needs to be done today.

Sometimes, based on the personality of their resident, a spouse or family will decide to say that the nursing home is a "temporary" placement when it is actually long-term. This is usually because that resident gets depressed, agitated, or angry and needs a goal they can aspire to. At other times it is not the resident who cannot accept long-term care; it is the spouse or family who cannot accept it and cannot tell their loved one the truth. In these situations, the family will tell their loved one they need to live in the nursing home "for the time being" or "until their health improves," and so forth. For this group of residents and families, this approach seems to help them; while in reality the resident is living long-term in a facility.

What about the others, though? *What happens if the resident finds out they have been "deceived," and their new, "for the time being" nursing home is actually a permanent placement?*

For those residents who continue to decline, it becomes readily apparent they cannot return home, and they will come to accept their new home.

For others who are still alert and oriented – and possibly still in denial of their situation – their first reaction will probably be anger. But this too passes because the spouse and family finally have to be honest about the situation, and the resident reluctantly realizes the nursing home is now their home.

Some residents, however, may fall into depression at the news since their own worst case scenario is now a fact. If this occurs, then professional consultation is best.

And for some residents who long ago accepted the nursing home as their "home," it may be their spouses and family who have to "catch up" to their loved one's unspoken understanding and acceptance.

> The ultimate lesson all of us have to learn is unconditional love, which includes not only others but ourselves as well.
> ~ Elizabeth Kubler-Ross

Time-Tested Tips

- Make an honest assessment of your loved one's heath and ability to function.

- What does the infirmed person need? Make a list. *Be specific.*

- Can you provide the care and assistance they need? *Be honest with yourself.*

- Determine whether your loved one's placement will be long-term or temporary.

- What is your guilt saying to you? What do others expect you to do? What do you expect of yourself?

- What is your conscious choice? Is this a non-negotiable choice?

    o To manage your guilt and prepare yourself to tell your loved one they will be staying in the nursing home, follow these four steps:

    o *Breathe.* Do the 4 - 4 Breathing technique to relax your mind-body and open yourself to new possibilities. Do it as often as you need to, and do it even more than you think you need to.

    o *State your choice to yourself.* This assumes you have clearly outlined the choices like we did with Lucy. If you haven't, go back and do this step so you can make a clear, conscious choice.

- o *Remind yourself of the reason(s) why you made that choice.*

- o *Repeat whenever the guilt pattern comes up.*

- Before speaking to your loved one, write out what you want to say. Keep it short and to the point, in plain language to help their understanding. Always include something about their medical condition since that reminds them of the reality of their situation and it may help them accept your conscious choice.

- **Practice Conscious Breathing every day:** Inhale deep…Exhale long. Repeat as often as you can.

> I am of the nature to grow old.
> There is no way to escape growing old.
> I am of the nature to have ill health.
> There is no way to escape ill health.
> I am of the nature to die.
> There is no way to escape death.
> All that is dear to me and everyone I love
> are of the nature to change.
> My actions are my only true belongings.
> I cannot escape the consequences of my actions.
> My actions are the ground on which I stand.
> ~ Buddha

Chapter 7
Reframing the Nursing Home Experience

"In here I'm sixteen, but this won't go!" Elsie snorted, poking at her chest, and then rattling her walker.

Elsie had been living at an Assisted Living Facility (ALF) following a rehab stay for a hip fracture, but still couldn't fathom why her body no longer worked the way it had for over ninety years. Elsie longed to return home and to her garden, but that was impossible since she lived alone and had no one to help her.

When she fell, Elsie spent two days on the bathroom floor until a neighbor called 911 saying they hadn't seen her as usual. The Fire Department broke into her house and found her on the floor, confused and dehydrated, unable to move due to her broken hip.

One day Elsie managed to walk out of the ALF and continued walking until the police found her several hours later and two miles away, hobbling over a bridge with her walker. Elsie didn't have a clue where she was or where she was going; she simply wanted to get back to the life she once knew and loved.

Brimming with feisty independence and frustration, Elsie had hit the proverbial nail on its head with her comment. In her mind she was still sixteen, full of plans and ideas, eager to get back to her springtime gardening, but her body refused to cooperate. The mind is timeless and perennially young; it cannot understand that the body has aged, become sick or injured, and can no longer do what it once was able to do so easily. Our minds also tend to follow our early programming and habits without much thought or reflection, assuming we wield control over life, including our bodies, when we actually have little power or control.

As a result, the mind can easily get stuck in a "time warp" where we believe that our experience and memories are the true, ongoing reality unless we go within and challenge the mind's assumptions and actively re-educate it. We find it difficult to accept the elemental fact that having a human body with all its incredible gifts, complexity, boundless energy and healing capability is subject to change, limitation, decline, and eventual decay. No one has figured out how to stop that progression. It's part and parcel of our experience and journey of being human.

Undaunted by the reality that her hip was still healing as well as her change in circumstances, Elsie tried to leave the ALF again. She had to be transferred to the nursing home next door since the Assisted Living was not a secured facility with locked doors.

Let's follow Elsie for a bit as she attempted to adjust to the nursing home and long-term care, something she'd vowed would never happen to her.

> The great secret that all old people share is that you really haven't changed in seventy or eighty years. Your body changes, but you don't change at all. And that, of course, causes great confusion.
> ~ Doris Lessing

Anywhere You Hang Your Hat

"I hate this. I want to go home. Why can't I go home?" Elsie asked repeatedly, never accepting anyone's answer because it wasn't what she wanted to hear. The nurses tried to explain her medical condition, but Elsie wasn't having any of it: She tried to leave the nursing home whenever they were busy, resulting in an exit-alarm anklet she had to wear. Her mind was laser focused on only one thing – going home, and that meant the home she had lived in for over fifty years. This was probably due to Elsie's increasing dementia following her hip surgery as well as her steadfast belief that home could only mean one place despite the passage of time and her declining health.

Every week, Elsie grew more depressed. At times she was agitated and angry, and even began refusing her medications or assistance with her everyday care. If anyone asked her what was wrong, she'd always answer, "I want to go home. This isn't my home." In addition, Elsie stopped eating, and began refusing showers and medications. Something had to be done.

What would you do when undeniable medical facts and basic reasoning are not changing someone's attitude so they are able to accept long-term placement?

What would you do when a resident is increasingly miserable, depressed, and uncooperative, and beginning to jeopardize their own welfare?

When going home is no longer an option for someone like Elsie, what options are there?

Certainly we could consider anti-depressant medication, as this could level out her mood. But potential side-effects and interaction with other mediations must be taken into consideration, especially at Elsie's advanced age.

Yes, Elsie could be transferred to another nursing home. But from all accounts that didn't seem a viable solution that would change her mind or improve her mood and attitude.

Here's what happened to Elsie. At their wit's end, the nursing home staff and Medical Director called for a psychological consult prior to prescribing anti-depressants. As is often the case with a resident like Elsie, the nurses warned me that she "wasn't talking to anyone." Although "hope may spring eternal," the hard reality of Elsie's mindset was that the odds were against any of us helping Elsie because Elsie didn't seem open to another perspective.

"I hate this," Else announced when we spoke. She jerked her head toward the hallway, disgust contorting her face. "The only way this can get better is for them to let me go home. Can you get me out of here?"

"No, I'm sorry. I don't have that authority," I answered truthfully.

"Then there's nothing to talk about." Elsie looked away, squeezing her lips, probably expecting me to leave quietly and let her be. But I wasn't about to give up so easily and I tried another line of approach.

"What's making you so unhappy today?"

No response from Elsie…except her lips tightened into a line.

"Maybe we can make things a little better for you while your hip continues to heal?"

I didn't tell Elsie she would be in nursing home "for the rest of her life" because that would have probably set off her anger and immediately ended our chance for a reasonable conversation. Instead, I was trying to get Elsie to talk a bit, so that once we reached a somewhat friendly footing I could reach out to her to see if we could then find some way to ease her distress, or at least make her feel as if someone understood her plight.

No response.

"Do you feel like you're a prisoner here?"

Elsie's eyes slid toward me, and she slowly nodded.

"Lots of people feel that way. They don't care what their medical problem is or what the doctors say. They want to go home. Like the old saying goes, "Home is where the heart is," and it isn't here," I responded sympathetically.

Tears welled up in Elsie's eyes as she nodded again.

We had finally made a connection, and at some level Elsie knew I wasn't trying to force her to accept the unacceptable. From there I asked her about her life and what she missed as well as what she didn't like in the nursing home. We came up with a couple of things that could be changed, such as ensuring that only female aides helped her. Elsie had been a widow for many years and was uncomfortable with a man helping her toilet or shower; it was something she hadn't encountered during her stay in the rehab unit or ALF. A staff change was instituted immediately which made Elsie feel a little calmer, and probably also safer. This raised her trust and confidence in me as someone who could help her – and without her knowing it, her trust in the "hated" nursing home also improved.

"It begins up here." – Reframing the Experience

Through the years I've learned to introduce small ways to reframe or view the nursing home experience differently, gauging what the resident accepts or refuses so I can modify my approach. At times I use their religious beliefs as a guideline, if those are important to them. I also tell new residents the stories of others, including a few who have spent thirty to forty years in nursing home. Elsie, like most people, was shocked at this news. "How can anybody spend forty years in a nursing home?" she asked.

I told her that extended placement is usually the result of a congenital problem or a subsequent medical condition or injury that, although serious and debilitating, is not terminal, and yet family or other institutions cannot care for the individual. The most interesting feature is that these long-term residents somehow managed to accept and be content while living in a nursing home. Some might say these residents were "resigned" to their situation – and they might be right – but most of these residents were definitely content and not severely depressed. I wouldn't say these residents are "happy" since that is characterized by a high level of cheerfulness and positive feelings where we feel all our needs and wants are satisfied.

I've ask the more alert of these long-term residents how they became content living in a nursing facility. "How did they make it their home?" As a rule, their answers coincided with what one woman who still had all her faculties told me.

"It begins up here," she said, and tapped her head. "One day I made up my mind the nursing home is my home. From that day, it got easier."

Elsie's response?

"Hell no, this ain't my home and never will be!"

I don't argue with the resident, I simply accept their answer and move on.

The mistake family and staff often make is to try to change the resident's mind by telling them how they're wrong, or that they should think and feel the way they want them to. This approach never works since a power struggle quickly develops. Some residents – like strong-minded Elsie – will fight back and refuse to consider even the sagest advice on principle. Others will nod and seem to agree, but they'll show their independence and contrariness in other, more indirect ways. In the end the resident wars against the nursing home with unsolvable complaints and accusations, and this ongoing struggle never leads to greater peace or physical comfort in the last chapter of their lives.

Instead of verbal warfare, I might ask the resident a few questions if they're open to some dialog. I invite their feedback on, "What do you think she meant when she said she made up her mind and made the nursing home her home?" Or, "Why would that woman make such a statement?" Or, "How can a nursing home be a 'home' for someone?"

These types of questions are impersonal since the focus is *on someone else or an abstract idea*. Yet, these questions also make the new resident think a little, broadening their belief of what "home" means. It also introduces a new idea that they had not considered: that someone can make another choice – a different choice, from them – regarding a nursing home. That's all I'm aiming for: *a different perspective where the resident might see, perhaps for the first time, how the nursing home can provide something of value to someone in their position.*

Sometimes I suggest that the resident consider viewing the

nursing home as their "second home" until their health improves and they are able to return home. For some this is more palatable than seeing the nursing home as "their (permanent) home." Either way, they still end up feeling more at peace in the facility with less symptoms and less acting-out behaviors that interfere with their care and well-being.

For a few, we might discuss what "home" means and whether it is a place we've gotten used to and feel comfortable in or whether it's more of a state of mind. After all, by the time they have arrived in a nursing home, all residents have lived in multiple homes – some more to their liking that others, but "home" nonetheless. Some residents may have moved more often and had to adapt to different living circumstances, and this makes adjustment to a nursing home easier, at least theoretically. But if some residents can feel at home in a nursing home, then it's possible that all of us could feel at home and at peace in a nursing home. It does, however, begin with acceptance of the basic fact that our health and body have deteriorated and we need a lot of assistance to get through the day and manage our health, even our survival.

For some residents, I may share a little of my father's experience in order to make the issue real and offset their thinking that I'm spouting unrealistic, "pie in the sky" psychobabble. So I tell them that my father accepted the fact that he had to live in the facility since there was no other option. It was not what he wanted or what I wanted, but there was no other choice given his health.

I explain that I also suggested to my dad it might be good if he got out of his room every day, and that he attend some of the daily activities the home offered to see if he liked any. He did that, and become active in the life of the nursing home, attending two or three activities every day, joining outings, painting (something he had never done), and becoming a Bingo regular (and he'd always hated Bingo). In so doing, my father began enjoying his new life as well as making relationships with other residents and staff members I didn't realize he knew.

And then, Christmas came in the nursing home. My father rarely spoke of his childhood, but from the little I knew, it was filled with hard times and little love, his younger brother the apple of his parent's eyes. He had to leave school and work as a child, to earn what he could in his downtrodden 1930s Havana neighborhood. Depression-era Christmas holidays filled with gifts and good times was not something he grew up with, and to me he never seemed interested in holidays. His nursing home, however, always made sure December was filled with holiday activities – and every resident received several gifts.

That first year, I saw my reserved father open up and enjoy the home's Christmas activities. He even began singing carols, which he'd never done before. He would smile broadly when he showed me the gifts he'd received, his delight obvious and contagious. Love and good cheer surrounded him in the nursing home, where he was loved for who he was and not for what he could do or did.

Unbeknownst to the staff, they were slowly healing his childhood wounds – and for that I'll be eternally grateful.

And no, he didn't receive special attention or accommodation because he was the father of the facility's psychologist. In fact, many staffers did not realize he was my father until much later. Through the years I've seen many residents be given the same kind of personalized attention, love, and validation of their unique worth simply because they are who they are and under the care of the nursing home's staff.

My father had, over time, done precisely what the woman I mentioned earlier had done: He had made the nursing home his home, and in so doing he was able to find peace and contentment in his final years.

One way this showed itself is whenever we'd go to his favorite restaurant, he'd often tell me when it was time to "go home," back to the nursing home. And when we turned into the facility's entrance, he'd smile and visibly relax, glad to be "back home." This reaction is not unique to my father: Many long-term residents will exhibit the same response especially after they leave the nursing home for a hospitalization, medical testing, or a doctor's appointment. Sometimes their reaction surprises even themselves, as they unexpectedly realize how much the nursing home has become their refuge and safe haven.

And Elsie? In time, she also became more comfortable living in the nursing home as she accepted the fact that her health had gone downhill and she needed assistance. She no longer fussed, argued with the staff, or refused her medications. Even her health improved! True to her nature, however, Elsie never called the nursing home her "home," even though it was.

> I'm going where a welcome mat is
> No matter where that is
> 'Cause any place I hang my hat is home.
> ~ Mercer & Harlen

A Warehouse is Not a Home

Some say nursing homes are "drab warehouses" for the elderly, who are "simply waiting for death's bidding." They ask, "How can such an institution be any kind of a 'home,' or provide love and healing to its residents?

This perception is certainly understandable. If you walk through any nursing home, chances are you will see a row of infirmed residents sitting limply in their wheel-chairs, clothes stained by the day's pureed meals, and drool oozing out the side of their mouths. Most don't speak, and if they do, they seldom make sense or even remember their names. Around them the staff goes about their business or talking amongst themselves, rarely paying attention to anyone unless they need to, and often trying to discretely use their cell phones whenever they get the chance.

Or, you might have heard a litany of complaints from a resident or someone who has a parent in a nursing home, and pray you'll never find yourself old, sick, and in a nursing facility.

Truth be told: In almost any nursing home you will often find such a sad looking line up of residents, and yes, some nursing homes are old and dreary, the smell of bodily fluids seeping into the hallways. And yes, a nursing home, whether for-profit or non-profit, is a business that is at times staffed by people who are there only for the paycheck, the administration always scrambling for more reimbursement and profit. No nursing home is ever as good as their brochure or website would lead us to believe – and none are as caring and loving as any of us would prefer. Certainly no nursing home is or can be as good as one's as own home, assuming that said home is a healthy environment where we are lovingly cared for by family, caregivers, physicians, and/or other medical personnel.

Since the early 1990s I've worked in many different nursing homes and ALFs, including bare-bones, old-style buildings; upscale facilities in continuing care communities; non-profit, church affiliated and secular institutions; and ones owned by both large and small corporations. I've even worked in a couple where the owners were later found to be illegally siphoning off money that should have gone to patient care or even necessary repairs. There have even been a few I walked away from for one reason or another, and some I would never place a loved one in. On the other hand, there are also good nursing homes that provide good care, but never perfect care. Nor will they please every resident and family member all of the time.

I am certainly no Pollyanna about the reality of old-age decline and nursing home care, nor do I rationalize away abuse, neglect, or disrespect of any kind that can be found in nursing homes and ALFs. However, these facilities are a reality of modern life and will continue to be. So, instead of decrying the less than ideal long-term care situation or assuming "…it'll never happen to us," let's face the situation squarely and think about how we ourselves can handle it more effectively and humanely. *How can we help to improve the lives of the old and infirmed in these homes?*

Volunteering two hours a week at a facility makes a huge difference – yet there are few volunteers in nursing homes. Also, perhaps consider giving a small donation to the Activities Department of a nearby facility to help a resident without family or means get a haircut, or buy toiletries or clothes from a thrift shop. Collect quarters and give them to the nursing home for their Bingo games since every resident likes to win a little something. One local middle school makes Christmas boxes for residents, while a high school offers credit for volunteering in nursing homes. It doesn't take much to brighten or ease someone's day.

> Carry out a random act of kindness, with no
> expectation of reward, safe in the knowledge that one
> day someone might do the same for you.
> ~ Princess Diana

As to those residents lined up in the hallway, what's the point? Is that what the residents want? Maybe yes, if the residents like to be around people and activity. Or no, if the resident prefers the quiet solitude of their room. But have you ever realized that the line-up also allows the nursing staff to get residents out of bed to avoid bedsores, as well as look after a larger number of residents quickly?

Sometimes you'll see a resident sitting by a nurse in the nurses' station, and wonder what the purpose is. This is a humane way to keep a confused or demented resident out of trouble or distress. I've even seen the nurses provide an activity in order to keep a resident active and/or validate an important past activity. For example, nurses in one facility made up a dummy patient chart they gave to a female resident every night with a snack. The resident, a retired charge nurse who had worked nights for decades, "worked" on the chart for a couple of hours and then returned to bed without incident, something that was impossible beforehand. What at first glance seemed to be demeaning busy work was actually supporting and validating a resident's well-being and self-esteem.

It's important to remember that a nursing home is more than residents who are sick, debilitated, or demented (suffering from one of the dementias, not "crazy" or "insane"). It is a thriving community of many diverse individuals, each with their own unique history and personality. Each resident also has a variety of needs, whether physical, medical, social, or psychological.

So, if you visit a nursing home and see a group of residents lined up, looking forlorn and isolated, don't look away and hurry by, then complain they're being treated like objects and not human beings, or that the nursing home is a greedy warehouse. *Do* something, by volunteering or donating what you can. Or, instead of walking by, acknowledge that human being in a wheel-chair by making eye contact and following Dolly's wonderful advice.

> If you see someone without a smile, give them yours.
> ~ Dolly Pardon

Choosing a Nursing Home

It's best to be at least somewhat prepared when having to choose a nursing home for long-term care. Probably the easiest way is to acquaint yourself via the internet with what's available in, or close to, your home town or that of your elderly parents. Then, if you get an unexpected phone call from a hospital about your elderly loved one, you won't be at a complete loss as to where to begin and what issues you face and will need to resolve quickly.

The following list is a starting point if this is your first time dealing with a nursing home for long-term care. (Please note that the issues, or "choice points," assume there is more than one facility to choose from.)

- **Location**

Ideally, the nursing home should be near you so you are able to visit regularly and at different hours throughout the week or month.

If your loved one is forgetful, confused, or has tried to leave their home repeatedly, it's best to choose a location that is away from a busy street and whose main exit is supervised and easily visible.

If your loved one has advanced dementia and needs almost constant supervision, consider a "closed" memory or dementia unit which will have locked doors with trained staff and activities.

- **Physical Appearance of the Facility**

If possible, pick a facility that is light and airy as supposed to one with dark, drab colors and long hallways which will give more of a "warehouse" feel. Older buildings will have smaller rooms with only a sink and/or toilet with full bathrooms and showers in the hallways. Newer nursing homes will typically have larger rooms with in-room bathrooms (full, or toilet and sink).

Some newer facilities may have large common areas or dining with meals served from a limited buffet line.

- **Cleanliness**

Is the facility kept clean? Does it smell of urine or feces? Please know that smells are inevitable depending on the resident population, illnesses, diaper changes, medical treatments, and so forth. However, these smells should not be ongoing for extended periods of time.

Are the residents clean? (Don't look for spotlessness since they may have come from lunch and spilled drinks or food on their clothing.) Overall, are the residents who cannot take care of their personal hygiene well kept? Do they have body odor or long nails? Are the men unshaven, hair unwashed or needing a trim?

Are the rooms clean, fairly tidy, and not smelly? Are there bugs or ants crawling about? Are meal trays left for hours before they are picked up, leaving behind the smell of old food?

- **Staff and On-site Services**

Visit the nursing home at different times of the day or week so you can get a feel for the facility, its staff, and how it runs. Weekends and nights will usually be quiet with a reduced staff.

Find out if the facility uses nursing staff from agencies on a regular basis, as this results in staff who do not know residents, and may have little investment in their care and well-being. While it is not usual for facilities to use agency staff to cover gaps in staffing, this should not be a major source of staffing for extended periods.

Ask if there are long-term staffers? Nursing, including both nurses and aides, typically exhibit a high turnover rate. Nevertheless, I prefer to see a core group of staffers who have been working in a facility for years since that gives the nursing home more stability and usually a better sense of caring for the residents.

As for the nurses and aides (CNAs), do they seem to be doing their job or slacking off? Do they seem interested in the residents or is there a pervasive "don't care" attitude? Are they adequately supervised? Are they respectful and courteous? They should not be using their cell phones, but you will see this behavior whenever they think they can get away with it.

Is the Medical Director on-site, or do they come to the facility? If so, how often? A few facilities have full-time Medical Directors on-site; most do not. Even so, find out if the physician(s) and/or their nurse practitioners (NP or ARNP) or assistants (PA) visit regularly. Do you have a choice of attending physician? Do any specialists come to the facility?

What ancillary services are available on-site? (Dental, Vision, Podiatry, Hearing, hairdresser, etc.) Is transportation provided or available? What is the cost, if any?

- **Don't expect perfection.**

Be aware of your expectations so you can gauge whether you are expecting too much and whether the facility can truly meet your standards as well as the needs of your loved one. Don't get caught in the trap of thinking what "should" happen as opposed to what is available in America's healthcare at this point in time. This is not a planet of perfection, and healthcare is just as imperfect as every other aspect of life. (This is not to say you ought to accept abuse, neglect, or disrespect.)

Be aware that nursing homes will typically say they can meet all your requests and needs. Maybe yes, but most likely not.

- **What are the needs and preferences of your loved one, especially when it comes to room choice?**

What are their personality tendencies? Be as specific as possible.

Even though they may have changed because of age, illness and/or dementia, in general, what are they like? For example, do they prefer solitude or do they get lonely and confused if they're alone too much or down a hallway? If they're shy and not talkative, chances are they will not like a talkative roommate or a loud TV. If they dislike sports, a roommate who watches televised sports all day long will be problematic for them. Others like and need to be close to the nurses' station so they are near people and activity.

What are their physical needs? Can their wheel-chair be rolled next to their bed in the facility? A resident should be able to maneuver their wheelchair or walker easily into the bathroom. If, for example, they have left-sided paralysis from a stroke, is there a grab bar on their right next to the commode?

Consider their beds carefully. Do they need a specific mattress: firm, soft, or air? Are they light sleepers? If yes, they'll need a quiet room. Some may prefer a "door bed" so they can watch activity outside, and leave their room easily. Another may prefer a "window bed" so they don't feel hemmed in, or can look out at nature or street activity.

Do they have room temperature preferences? Some prefer a cold room, especially those with respiratory illnesses and MS, while others prefer a warm or even a hot room.

Are there any hearing or vision impairments? What accommodations, if any, are available?

What is the overall resident mix? For example, if your loved one has little cognitive decline, they may not like to be in close proximity to more demented residents who may wander into their rooms, handle or take items, lay down in their bed, cry out, moan or curse for no apparent reason, or even attempt to undress. Some new residents do not like to be around obviously sick and disabled individuals, which they will encounter in any nursing home.

It's impossible to specify all the preferences and needs your loved one has, especially if you have had little direct contact with them over the years. As they live in the nursing home, some of these will become evident and sometimes a room change is needed. To begin, do your best, and try to be as practical as possible. It will not be perfect.

Some residents prefer or would do better in a private room,

but these entail extra cost since third party payers like Medicaid will not pay for private rooms. However, some newer facilities may have a room design called "shared entry," with a partial wall separating each side, or single rooms with shared bathrooms that provide greater privacy.

- **Check out the nursing home's reputation in the community.**

This information, as well as annual State surveys and ratings, can be found on the internet. The facility should be able to provide you with their latest State survey. In addition, check with the State's Health Department or whatever department oversees nursing homes and read their ratings.

Keep in mind, however, that State surveys reflect a snapshot of a facility as it compares with written standards. A citation for a failing or "deficiency" may not be as significant as it looks on paper. For example, once during a State survey I saw a long-term resident in a wheel-chair blow his nose and immediately tuck the tissue behind a railing. A surveyor was walking some fifteen feet behind him and citied the facility even though it was not possible for anyone to dispose of that used tissue in that short amount of time.

If you do read a State survey, it will typically look at key areas such as Quality of Care, Quality of Life, Safety, Staffing Patterns (to ensure they comply with State required minimums), Dietary, etc. You will see deficiencies as well as proposed remedies and follow-up surveys. Try to tease out genuine care issues and noncompliance from incomplete paperwork. Nursing homes and their staff have an enormous amount of written documentation they must do, and the amount and complexity seems to grow with every passing year even with computerized documentation systems.

If you get the chance, speak to other family members or "alert and oriented" residents (or as some residents say, those who still have "all their marbles"). There will always be complaints, but are they in the distant past, ongoing, or one time? Are you hearing the same complaint over and over again? If you are, that may point to a real problem as opposed to the more common complaints and "lack of perfection" in nursing home services. To get a balanced perspective, try to speak to residents and families who are satisfied, assuming you are not intruding upon their privacy.

Remember, even the best nursing homes are not perfect, and residents will typically complain that they have to "wait too long" for an aide or nurse. It should never be an hour unless there is a major emergency in the unit, nor should a resident remain in wet diapers overnight (this can lead to sores), and so forth. Also, aides should not come into a room and turn off the call light without helping the resident, although this happens. If any of this occurs or happens repeatedly, speak to the Unit or Nurse Manager, Director of Nursing, or Administrator.

- **Finances**

This will need to be addressed up front with the Business Office, including third party insurance, Social Security and/or pension payments. If the resident will be "private pay," meaning they are paying the nursing home, there will probably be other charges such as non-covered medications, supplies, transportation to/from doctor's visits, and such. Try to get as clear a picture of the costs involved so you can to avoid unpleasant surprises as well as effectively plan for your loved one's care. Financial management will take time as you learn how the system works in your loved one's particular case.

Lastly, if the first nursing home doesn't work out as you hoped, consider a transfer to another facility. A marathon of misery leads nowhere, and the goal is to have as peaceful a nursing home experience as humanly possible. Consult the Long-term Care Checklist in the Appendix to see if any of those care issues apply to your loved one at this point in their life.

> Too often we underestimate the power of a touch, a smile, a kind word, a listening ear, an honest compliment, or the smallest act of caring, all of which have the potential to turn a life around.
> ~ Leo Buscaglia

Complaints, Complaints, and More Complaints

Complaints from residents are plentiful, often repetitive, and once in a great while creative and unique. Some complaints can be remedied, even immediately, and some can never be fixed even in the best of nursing homes. Moreover, some complaints reflect the primary underlying issue every resident faces, which can be summed up as: "Getting too old in a sick and disabled body and then having life change in ways nobody likes and can control." Unfortunately, this is a problem that cannot be solved. There is no perfection in life despite our most ardent needs, desires, expectations, and "shoulds." Deep down we all know and share this basic truth, but few accept it completely and without reservation, especially when life does not go our way and our body is weak and hurts in one way or another.

Below are the most common areas of complaints followed by a discussion how the responsible family member/care manager can better understand and address these issues. Bear in mind if the resident is "their own person," meaning they are legally competent and make their own decisions, the care manager's role is often limited. The four main areas of criticism and grievances are:

- Aides or Certified Nursing Assistants (CNAs) not providing the help your loved one wants or needs in the way they prefer or in a timely manner;

- Roommates and/or the characteristics of their room; or even the physical features of a facility;

- Food and Laundry; and

- Miscellaneous, including Activities as well as the ever present Loss of Autonomy, Independence and Freedom.

Complaints about the Aides (CNAs)

From the point of view of the resident's daily life and satisfaction, the most important staff member in a long-term care facility is the resident's **aide or CNA** (a position that years ago used to be called an "orderly"). This person is also the least trained and lowest paid in the nursing department. In Florida, for example, an aide undergoes a few weeks training and thus knows little of the medical, rehab, dietary, social, or psychological aspects of their residents or yet alone the State regulations which govern every aspect of a nursing home.

Aides provide daily care and assistance to some of the residents, such as bathing, dressing, toileting, bringing meals, and feeding. If they are trying to do a good job, they are typically quite busy, and along with the nurses may stay past their shift if they need to finish some documentation.

Being a CNA is not an easy job. The residents may not like to be told what to do or be comfortable with others providing personal care to them, and in response some will hit, kick, pinch, swat away, spit, curse, grab personal areas, make sexual comments or requests, or call aides names and racial epithets. CNAs are often not given their due and respect in terms of how important they are in a nursing home or what good, hard work they've been doing day in and day out. On the other hand, all it takes is one or a few "bad aides," something that makes the resident miserable and leads them to complain again and again.

Most residents cannot distinguish between an aide and a nurse, and think they are appropriately asking for medications or reporting a medical problem when they are not. The aide may not relay that request to the nurse or it is forgotten in the rush of going to help another resident in another room. This results in complaints that the staff is not addressing a medical issue or pain. This often happens regarding PRN medications (that require the resident to ask for them). The forgetful resident may not remember or know how to ask for pain meds, so the main issue then is that the request or problem was never brought to the attention of the appropriate staffer, in this case the nurse.

If your loved one complains that no one is helping them or bringing them pain medications, check if this dynamic is happening and whether the nurse knows of the problem. One easy way residents can identify their nurse is that he or she will be the one who gives them medications. (Nurses do much more than give medications, but this is a concrete way for a resident to identify their nurse.) Some facilities will have staff wear different colors to signify their department, but residents may still not understand or remember the color scheme. Further compounding the problem is that the resident will have multiple aides and nurses throughout the week, so they cannot keep track of who is who.

An aide that is attentive, considerate, and courteous will make the resident's life easier and more tolerable or satisfactory. A good aide will take the time to know the resident and modify their approach based on what works best and causes the least pain and discomfort. But if an aide is rough, rude, unkind, lazy, uncaring, bullying, does only the minimum or is always in a hurry, or speaks too quickly, too softly or with a heavy accent (which is difficult for the elderly and hearing impaired to understand), that will result in multiple complaints and distress even if there is no abuse or neglect. Unfortunately, not enough good aides exist to fill all the available job openings.

A good aide may well become your resident's friend or even feel like family, especially if there is a long-term relationship. Such an aide can also provide valuable information as to how your loved one is doing, whether they are declining or experiencing other problems, or even if they need underwear, toiletries, etc. Keep in mind that a good aide will have "bad days" or hurried interactions; it happens to all of us. Some residents will be aware of this and let a complaint go after they've vented their frustration.

If at all possible, I recommend that you *get to know your resident's care team*, i.e., the nurse and aide for every shift, including weekends, *and develop a congenial working relationship with them*. Through the years I've found that if a resident is exhibiting a problem behavior, there will usually be a CNA who doesn't have difficulty with that resident. This is because those CNAs are approaching the resident differently or have a better understanding and tolerance for them. It pays off to seek those aides out and learn from them.

If your resident does have a good aide, please compliment the aide and/or tell their supervisors. They receive many, many complaints, but seldom gratitude for a job well done. For example, a Spanish speaking resident who had forgotten her English and initially was paranoid and difficult, finally began to calm down and adjust to long-term care. One afternoon she reported with a big smile that earlier that day she had "a great shower." It made her feel so good that it made her day. When I spoke to her aide, at first she tightened up expecting a complaint, but when she heard the compliment, she too had a big smile. It made her day, and probably paved the way for more good days for both of them.

Refrain from tipping since most facilities do not allow this, and if a CNA is caught accepting a tip, they may lose their job. If your resident or you wish to give an aide a "thank you" gift, especially during the holidays, please ask the nurse, social worker or other manager if this is allowed.

Many residents fear that the aide and/or their colleagues will retaliate somehow if they are reported and so do not want a complaint to be made on their behalf. Unfortunately, retaliation or "payback" has been known to happen, including slowness in responding to call lights, so this is not a wholly unfounded fear. *As a family member, you need to be aware of this possibility so your resident does not pay the price, even if it's with needless worry and anxiety.* Some residents say they want to "solve the issue themselves," and it's best to allow them to do so because then they feel empowered and more comfortable in their home with their care team.

If you do need to **report a problem or complaint**, be as specific as possible providing concrete details and examples. The usual recommendation is to go up the "chain of command" beginning with the resident's aide or the person directly involved with your resident's care and the issue. However, it may not be possible to speak to that aide if they are on a different shift from when you visit or they are an on-call agency CNA, or if your resident cannot provide a name or details so they can be identified. For example, for a lost item of clothing, the Laundry staff would probably be first choice although the aide, nurse, or social worker are often the ones contacted.

Next up the chain is your resident's nurse, who is probably not comfortable with supervising or setting limits with aides, and will usually focus solely on her nursing responsibilities. The next level up is Unit or Nurse Manager, then the social worker, Director of Nursing, and lastly, the Administrator or Executive Director of the facility.

The person to whom you address complaints will vary according to the nature of the complaint, and going up the "chain of command" isn't always the most productive. If it's a minor problem and related to ongoing routine such as dressing habits, then speaking directly to the resident's aide might work well. If the issue is nursing care, pain, wounds, or medications, the nurse is the one to speak to and they will contact the attending physician if needed. But if the issue is rough care, lack of assistance, answering call lights by turning them off and walking out, taking a long time to answer a call light or bathroom light, and/or disrespect or inappropriate language as well as potential abuse, then a manager should be brought into the situation.

When making a complaint, **be specific by providing these facts:**

- *Who was involved? Can they be identified somehow?*

- *What happened?* Give concrete details that describe what happened or what the aide did or did not do (as opposed to labeling the behavior). Your words need to "paint a picture" so that someone who was not present can visualize the behavior and the incident. (See the example below.) *Did it happen once or is the problem ongoing?*

- *What was said?* (Actual verbatim quotes are best if you have them.)

- *When did the problem occur?* Day and time or shift are needed so an aide is not wrongly accused and reprimanded.

- *Where did it occur? Are there any witnesses?*

Be accurate. Don't exaggerate or overstate your case, or become overly emotional or angry. Don't intimidate or threaten. Vague, over-generalized complaints such as "The aides are rude," without some identifying information are basically impossible to track down and correct.

For example, if the complaint is expressed as, "The aides are rude," then is the problem with *all* the aides, or only one aide? What does the resident or family member mean by "rude?" (Rudeness can vary greatly from one person to the next, one generation to the next.)

On the other hand, if a female resident says, "Last night, my aide told me to "Wash my p****" when she took me to the bathroom," this is specific enough that the Nurse Manager can address it. This will help the manager address the problem effectively, which usually begins by speaking to the aide and educating them. If abuse is suspected, the aide is usually suspended while an investigation ensues in keeping with facility and State policy.

In the event there is no improvement, proceed up the chain of command to the Administrator and beyond if needed. However, remember to prioritize complaints and care issues according to how important they are, so it is not a list of petty annoyances or demands. For instance, I've heard complaints from some residents that an aide "refused to help them." But when questioned further, the resident expected the aide to come quickly for minor things the resident could do, such as hand them an item off their rolling table which they could easily reach, water their plants and flowers, or hand-wash certain items (not part of an aide's job), and so forth. Furthermore, in a nursing home the general rule is for residents to be as independent as possible, and do for themselves. So if an aide actually fulfills these types of requests, they're undermining the resident's abilities and reinforcing unreasonable expectations.

In one facility, for example, three residents complained about one aide's manner. But in the recent past they had all reported she was a "good aide" and was "never rough" or "left things undone." These complaints didn't make sense, so I asked them for examples so I could see the problem in my mind's eye. It turned out that what they wanted was for the aide to be more friendly and talkative. This young aide was shy and usually said very little, but they liked her and wanted more contact. In this instance, a little education and encouragement by the Nurse Manager went a long way to improve what was already a good working relationship between an aide and her residents.

Repetitive minor, even petty complaints will not foster a good working relationship with any staff, and may well reinforce a demanding or imperial attitude on the part of some residents. I've seen some residents treat aides as if they are personal servants, snapping their fingers and expecting immediate attention. This attitude and behavior is not appropriate in any healthcare situation and will not enhance any relationship.

Also, keep in mind that residents have lots of time on their hands and can become overly focused on details and imperfections. Furthermore, they did not choose to live in a nursing home voluntarily, and often feel as if they lost their life as well as their independence and self-esteem. As a result, they are liable to vent their ongoing frustration in some way. For example, they may criticize aides because things are not done the way the resident would have done them in their own home.

Consequently, family members may receive a litany of stored-up complaints and frustrations from these residents. This does not mean these grievances are vitally important or solvable. For better and for worse, the residents are living in a healthcare institution due to their compromised health, and so things are not as they are at home. Nor does this kind of complaining indicate that family must fix the situation as if by magic. Moreover, the resident may be venting to: Let you know they are unhappy with the placement on principle; make you feel bad or guilty for their plight and for putting them in the facility; or get you to take them home. And if the resident suffers from dementia or other cognitive impairment, their complaints may be from the past and may even have been already resolved; may be inaccurate, vague or pejorative; or may be a reflection of the dementia process rather than ongoing reality.

One simple way to help determine or prioritize how important a resident's complaint is to ask yourself, "How important is their complaint on a one-to-ten scale? How important is it to their health and well-being?"

On this scale, ten signifies life or death, like the beginning of a stroke that means we need to get to an emergency room right now. Eight or nine indicates close to life or death, like fainting; losing consciousness momentarily; severe, debilitating pain; or an oozing wound that will likely get worse without medical attention. One signifies not important at all, like a passing annoyance such as lukewarm coffee or too many pieces of bacon on the breakfast tray. Respond in accordance to the importance of the complaint – and sometimes that will mean you are going to let a low number complaint slide by.

Sometimes the CNA, nurse or other staff member may complain about your resident. Then what do you do? Do you condemn, scold or "chew out" your loved one, or do you let it go and hope the behavior doesn't repeat? Truth is, there are no clear-cut rules that apply to all situations over the course of your loved one's placement and continued decline.

With both my father and the residents I counsel, I follow the basic guidelines outlined above to determine the details and importance of the complaint, and whether it merits a heart-to-heart discussion with the resident. Bear in mind that like residents, staff sometimes need to vent if they've been having a difficult time with a resident they can never please, and they may need a helping hand from you. So what you should first do is simply listen; they're people too, and they are doing a demanding job. After giving the staff my attention, I usually ask what they would like to see improve, and this helps both of us figure out whether it's even possible, given the resident, their health status, and primary personality traits.

> God, grant me the serenity to accept the things I cannot change,
> The courage to change the things I can,
> And the wisdom to know the difference.
> ~ Serenity Prayer

One common complaint is along the lines of "There aren't enough aides. Why don't they hire more aides?" What residents and families do not realize is that nursing homes are staffed according to State guidelines, and if they meet those guidelines, then the nursing home is in compliance. Don't expect the facility to hire more aides above those guidelines; it won't happen.

In addition, staffing is affected by census (number of residents in the facility; seasonal fluctuations in census occur in places like Florida), and of course, "the budget." It takes an enormous amount of resources and staff to keep a nursing home operational. From the resident's perspective this is all irrelevant. Their issue is having to wait too long for help, or that the aides are in a rush and only do the minimum, or hurt them with rough handling. The better use of any increase in funds might be to train aides to elevate their professional and people skills – and then pay them accordingly.

In summary, if your resident complains or you notice something amiss:

1. Get the details or specifics;

2. Determine the complaint's importance or priority;

3. Decide whether to bring the concern to the attention of the immediate staff member(s) or to a manager;

4. Be aware of possible retaliation or "punishment" for reporting the complaint; and,

5. In the event of abuse or neglect, speak to the Nurse Manager or other available manager immediately.

How do I, as the psychologist, handle resident complaints? First, if I decide to report a complaint, then I make sure to see how the facility responded to the genuine problem. If, for example, I bring an important care issue, such as uncontrolled pain or crude language to the attention of a manager, I expect follow through in a timely fashion. This may not mean a solution that the resident and/or their family likes and approves of, or one that solves the issue for all time. However, I do expect that the manager and/or resident will tell me the next time I see them that the issue was remedied, such as new pain meds or a change in scheduling that works better, or the cessation of crude language; or even a change in aides if that is the best solution.

Now, if I believe the issue that is brought up is more along the lines of unreasonable resident expectations, I focus on that aspect. If the resident likes or needs to vent, criticize, and complain, I let them do that for a time if that makes them feel better and more at peace in the facility. After all, every resident is there because of medical necessity, doesn't feel well, and are not at their best.

If a resident complains of rudeness, I inquire whether it's abuse, bad professional manners, the aide is having a "bad day," or if the resident is personalizing the aide's demeanor, mood, or personality. And, if the resident tells me not to report a complaint, I respect that assuming their well-being is not jeopardized. Nonetheless, I do ask about the issue in the future to ensure it is not a reoccurring or escalating problem.

As you can see, I prioritize complaints and problems as well as get basic, concrete details so if I do speak to a manager, they'll know this is something important and they have the information they need to begin their investigation. Although I always want every nursing home to offer a great healing and living environment, I realize the reality and limitations of modern day healthcare as well as the people who provide it.

What should you do when a facility and its staff, from the

aide to the Administrator, brushes away every complaint and problem, even if the resident's health is at risk? This shows the facility's true colors, and it might be time to involve the Ombudsman or the State – every facility should have contact information readily available. In addition, familiarize yourself with the resident's legal rights, and that includes transferring to another nursing home.

Roommates, Food, Laundry, and Activities

Roommates present a host of issues beginning with the fact that the elderly have typically not lived with roommates except for: their spouse; their siblings (back when they were young); or their military buddies (if they were in the military, and usually many decades ago). Hence, sharing a small space with a stranger can be challenging and off putting, especially since both are probably "set in their ways" and also do not feel well. Although most nursing homes try to pair the best combination possible, there is no way to predict who will hit it off, who will annoy one another, or who will dislike one another with a passion and want them out of the room or the facility.

Some roommates become friends, even buddies, while others argue and fuss at one another. One roommate might be forward, critical, or pushy, and tries to control the room and the roommate to get that what they want (such as the room all to themselves). Some residents complain their roommate "gets too much attention," while they receive less than what they want or feel they should get. And sometimes roommates have differing opinions about religion, politics, and so forth, and this can make the living situation uneasy, or even contentious, between them.

The main areas of roommate contention are: room temperature; television habits; room noise; and bathroom habits or time spent in the bathroom. Some residents prefer a room to be hot, even turning on the heat in summer, while others like a cold room with the AC running and blowing a breeze. Some watch TV all day, while others prefer silence or their own TV programs. If there are two televisions going, each with different programs and the volume turned up, there will be endless problems. A resident's need for sleep can be disturbed by a roommate's habit, such as late-night TV, getting up often to go to the bathroom, noisy nighttime care, or loud snoring.

Some residents spend a lot of time in the bathroom, oblivious to their roommate's needs. Some are messy and leave things about, while others are clean and tidy, their area clearly delineated with the expectation that their roommate will reciprocate. Some roommates may have medical issues such as a colostomy bag which requires changing that can be smelly and offensive to the other person in the room.

Sometimes family members request roommates for their resident who are social and talkative in the misguided idea that their loved one will enjoy having someone to chat with and who will be supportive. These families want this roommate to spark more conversation, social contact, and mental stimulation, and in so doing, dampen their loved one's isolation or depression. Please know this is *not* a roommate's job, and in fact places an undue burden on them. Roommates are not there to socialize or improve your loved one's life, and to think so dismisses the roommate's own illness, needs, and preferences.

On the other hand, sometimes a more alert resident can provide valuable information about your loved one to staff as well as family. For example, your loved one may complain bitterly about the aides, yet the roommate who has the same aide and may have witnessed the interactions can clarify what, if anything, was truly problematic or a valid grievance. Some roommates, however, do not wish to get involved or offer any information, and that must be respected.

Some roommates, however, believe that it is their job to care for and support a new roommate. They can sometimes become meddling and controlling, even offering unsolicited advice and intervening with nurses and aides. Some residents feel burdened by having a sicker roommate in the bed next to them, to the point they check on the roommate throughout the day and night. Some even attempt to help them get out of bed or into the bathroom. This is also not a roommate's job. If a resident gets paired with a needy or difficult individual, the result is one demands and the other feels beholden to do what they want.

Family and other visitors are sometimes noisy, or come in a group filling up half of the room. This sparks complaints by the other resident that the visitors are noisy or they can't get through to the bathroom easily, and so on.

Lastly, if your resident has a roommate or nearby neighbors with dementia, these residents may come into their room uninvited, stand and stare, rummage through closets and drawers, take items, get into an empty bed for a nap, yell or curse without provocation, smell due to wet or solid diapers or refusals to bathe, and so forth. Any roommate issues and problems should be brought to the attention of the social worker or Nurse Manager. If roommates are incompatible for whatever reason, the resident and/or their family can request a room change and this is often the best solution to incompatibility and conflict.

In a nursing home, **food** will be a source of ongoing complaints. On limited budgets, nursing homes must provide three meals a day plus snacks and nutritional supplements such as protein shakes. It is institutional food, not home cooking – and it never will be.

As a result, a resident's complaints range from food that is overcooked, dry or has too much gravy or sauce; the food is bland, too salty or unsalted; to meals with too much chicken or "mystery meat," not enough fresh fruits and vegetables, and few if any salads (not common since infirmed elderly don't seem to eat salads or are unable to do so). Often there may be too many sweets offered (true, since these typically are readily available), or "weird" food the resident doesn't know, has never cooked or eaten, and simply doesn't want to try. If the resident is on a restricted diet, such as "mechanical soft" (chopped) or pureed due to failed swallowing tests, the resident complains these meals "don't look right" and "don't taste good." But the doctor orders these special diets, something the aides and nurses cannot override without authorization.

In addition, if your resident eats in a dining room, they may complain if they are seated with someone who is a sloppy eater or has "bad" table manners. Or, in some situations, it's best for residents who do not get along with one another to move to another table.

Residents will also complain that the facility "throws away too much food," but the home doesn't have another choice due to health regulations. Lastly, if they've lived in the nursing home for a while and have tasted all their menus several times, they'll even start to complain about favorite dishes.

If at all possible, and to help reduce resident food complaints, bring in some food (small portions) to your resident; take them out to eat for a change of pace; or encourage them to ask for the alternate or a sandwich (which most facilities can provide on a limited basis). If you do bring in snacks, try to limit sweets or simple carbs, since these will affect sugar levels as well as mood and behavior. Also, encourage your loved one to limit their caffeine consumption depending on how it affects them. For any dietary issues, please speak to the nurse or dietician.

Another common area of complaints is **laundry,** with residents and families alike reporting missing, misplaced, stolen, or damages items. The typical nursing home does a truckload of laundry every day, which includes not only residents' clothing, but also linens, towels, kitchen and dining room items. It is no wonder items go missing or misplaced, sometimes later found in another's resident's closet or drawers. Clothing also gets stolen now and then, as well as damaged. Facilities use commercial dryers and these can damage, shrink or destroy clothing.

The rule of thumb I followed with my father was to never buy him expensive clothes, polo shirts or t-shirts that had to be put on over the head and shoulders (as this can hurt an old body). I always bought him elastic-waist athletic-style pants that were easy on/off and do not require a belt, as well as button-down cotton cardigans and vests (facilities can get cold and drafty). When an article of clothing went missing, I accepted that and moved on, restocking my father's wardrobe every so often. If a resident and their family needs to keep a tight rein on expenses, consider buying clothing at a good thrift shop. When you buy a resident a pair of shoes, make sure they are comfortable, probably wide, and have non-slip soles. And always, *refrain from buying expensive clothing, shoes, or jewelry, because sooner or later, something will disappear, or that pretty dress or shirt will get stained.*

Every nursing home has scheduled **Activities** throughout the week, though the frequency and quality can vary greatly among facilities. Some families and friends believe that all residents should attend activities, but this is unrealistic and does not take into account individual differences or health status. Some residents simply do not like group activities and prefer to remain in their rooms doing solitary activates. That is their right, and to cajole someone to socialize when they do not feel up to it or are loners by nature is both unkind and inconsiderate.

Suggest to your new resident that they attend some activities to see if any appeal to them, *but do not push them to attend*. Sometimes, however, even the most solitary of residents will enjoy music programs, church services or outings, and that ought to be encouraged if they feel well enough to attend.

> A population that does not take care of the elderly
> and of children and the young has no future, because
> it abuses both its memory and its promise.
> ~ Pope Francis

Loss of Freedom and Control

Every resident enters long-term care reluctantly and feels the sting of losing their independence and sense of self-sufficiency. They may have felt that they were managing life their way, and would be able do so until the day they died. With this comes a loss of self-esteem and identity, as well as loss of social contacts and friends, some of whom may have already died or moved away, and some who will never visit once a resident enters a nursing home.

Control over one's life is an elusive and overarching concept we all seem to value and desire, believing it is a necessary aspect of our existence. In reality, no one actually controls or can control their life as much as they want or imagine. But in a practical sense we all make choices and try to arrange our lives the way we prefer and according to what we've become accustomed to – and that passes for control.

The loss of control is felt more acutely for some residents than others, depending on their personality, history, and the need to avoid feeling they are at the mercy of others, or forces and situations they cannot influence. For some residents this triggers depression with its sadness and pessimism, or else they view the placement as a disgrace of some kind that signifies they are less a person or less an adult. Others adapt to this change rather quickly and can move forward, no longer burdened by having to try to control a life that has runway from them due to illness and old age.

For family members, it's important to be sensitive to these issues so we do not expect our resident to casually dismiss their losses and swiftly adjust to long-term care as we and the facility take over more and more of their lives. It is important to remember that it is a process that will take time and have its inevitable ups and downs. *If your resident is showing signs of deepening depression (see next chapter) or resistance to placement that is impacting their care, please discuss this with their nurse or social worker, and consider a consult with a mental health professional.*

> Eventually all things fall into place. Until then, laugh at
> the confusion, live for the moments, and know
> everything happens for a reason.
> ~ Albert Schweitzer

Time-Tested Tips

- What do you expect the nursing home to provide? Be specific.

  Can the nursing home meet your expectations? Your loved one's expectations? Are you or your loved one secretly expecting the nursing home to be perfect and thus make life easier and problem free?

- What does long-term care mean to you?

- What do you expect for your parents or your spouse in long-term care?

- Do you expect your resident to improve? In what ways? Can their health and functioning actually improve?

- Do you expect your resident to be happy? Nice? Considerate? Understanding? Are they able to do that? Are you expecting too quick an adjustment?

- If your resident has dementia, educate yourself what dementia is, and what their current level of functioning is. Given that, adjust your expectations. *Don't expect or demand the impossible.*

- When choosing a nursing home, remember it will never be perfect.

- There will be complaints from your resident or perhaps

even their aide(s); it's the nature of life and nursing home placement. Prioritize the complaints according to importance. If you plan to speak to staff or a manager about the more important complaints, try to get concrete details so you can describe what happened and what needs to change for the better. This will help the listener better understand the problem. It also points the way to how the problem can be remedied or lessened.

- Be mindful that your parent or spouse has lost a great deal of health and daily functioning in order to be placed in a nursing home. This loss includes their freedom, autonomy, sense of "controlling" or managing their own life, and even their privacy. In response, are you acting too "parental" toward them, and dictating their lives or how they should behave in the facility and with other residents?

- Before visiting your loved one in a nursing home, remind yourself they are old, infirmed, and in the last stage of life. If you feel stressed as you drive into the nursing home, do your breathing technique in the parking lot before walking in.

  During your visit, follow The Golden Rule and treat them with compassion and patience. Remember, one day you too will be old, and it maybe you who's living in a nursing home or ALF and waiting for a friendly face to come through the door.

- **4 - 4 Breathing:** Breathe in through the nose to a count of 4.
  Gently hold it for a count of 2.
  Then exhale through the mouth for a count of 4.
  Repeat at least three times.

Your task is not to seek for love, but merely to seek and find all the barriers within yourself that you have built against it.
~ Rumi

Chapter 8
From Depression to New Ways of Being

"Can't an old broad have a little fun?" Beverly huffed, completely exasperated with the nursing home and the State of Florida. "They should stay out of my business. At my age, I don't get many chances, you know?"

What could I say? Beverly was right from that point of view since she was nearing the end of her life and she knew it. But there were legal factors at work here, and they took precedence over desire.

For the past several months Beverly had been having a consensual sexual relationship with her nighttime nurse. He should have known better since sex between a healthcare professional and a patient is forbidden, even if the patient or resident consents knowingly and has the mental abilities to give informed consent (which Beverly possessed). Sexual relationships are legally forbidden because the patient does not have the same level of power and freedom of choice as the professional. Thus, the resident could easily be taken advantage of, and even if they're not, the end of the relationship would likely bring heartache no resident needs. Moreover, the professional's involvement could well color decision-making and medical care, both during and after the end of the affair, or lead to financial trickery and fraud.

"Since my Bobby died, I haven't been close to any man. It gets lonely here, and he (the nurse) and I didn't hurt anybody." Beverly gave me a sad, tired face, looking every bit of her eighty-five years. "What happens now? Will he lose his job?"

I nodded in response. Yes, he would lose his job as well as his nursing license, and possibly his marriage, but that was his business. My focus was on Beverly, who had been distraught since the affair came to light after the aide noticed something amiss and brought it to the attention of the administration. Thankfully, Beverly and the nurse readily admitted to their affair, curtailing the need for a stressful investigation.

Nonetheless, the State and Beverly's children were notified, and her children responded with respect and caring. No one wanted Beverly to suffer or feel guilty; she was close to death, and shaming or blaming her would serve no purpose. The goal was to make the situation as painless as possible for Beverly, who died peacefully a few months later. And like the classy, warm hearted lady she'd always been, Beverly requested that the nurse and his wife visit her so she could apologize to his wife in person. Beverly had never wanted to hurt her or interfere with their marriage, even though of course the affair did.

The Capacity for Consent

Sexual desire and the need for closeness and to be touched can continue well into our elder years, even though the body's ability to perform and respond changes and fades. Nursing home residents have the legal right to engage in sexual activity in nursing homes, but never with staff. This assumes compliance with three main factors which may be defined differently depending on the jurisdiction. Also, keep in mind the following is from a psychologist's point of view, and not that of a lawyer. These issues include:

1. The resident willingly consents or gives permission, and is not coerced nor coerces another resident;

2. The resident has the capacity to consent, and that means they know what they are about to do, possible consequences, and feel free to say "No" or otherwise decline; and,

3. Any sexual activity must be done so in private in order to respect the privacy of roommates and/or other residents.

In practice, issues regarding sexual activity and consent can quickly become thorny with no easy or clear-cut answers for the nursing home, medical staff, the resident's family or care manager. For example, if an elderly husband demands conjugal visits or climbs into bed with his demented and infirmed wife and she does not clearly say "No" or push him off, is that knowing consent on her part? What if she makes some protest the roommate hears, or the staff notices some physical consequences such as abrasions or infections; does this override apparent and nonverbal consent?

Some husbands have said their wife "smiled" or otherwise responded as if she liked the sexual stimulation, and that meant she gave consent. Is this enough? If a dementia resident can no longer speak or even respond to cognitive examination, there might be no way to know if she truly understands her husband's request or foreplay, and what it means at this point in her life. What can adult children do if they disagree with their father, and feel their mother's well-being is being compromised?

What if the husband does not have legal say over his wife, but instead someone else has Power of Attorney (POA) or Guardianship? What is the nursing home supposed to do if he and/or the resident press for conjugal visits?

It's clear that when it comes to sex in our later years in a facility, there are multiple legal issues involved, which the States may define and handle differently. Here are several examples to highlight some of these issues.

A ninety-two-year-old female resident was caught in his act of giving oral sex to a ninety-three-year-old resident with a severe heart condition. Much like Beverly, they both said they "liked it," and clearly they were old enough to make their decisions. Moreover, since their spouses were long since dead and they "weren't hurting anyone," what was the problem? The problem here was that the man's three daughters were outraged and would not accept their father having sexual relations with anyone other than their mother. In addition, the daughters, who held Durable POA status, were worried this activity might trigger another heart attack, and they wanted it stopped immediately. However, lawyers tell me that a POA cannot override if a person is competent. In order to maintain peace and not cause future medical problems, the staff finally told the female resident she could not visit him in his room any longer.

Another elderly couple, both widowed with early dementia, became friendly in their ALF and continued their relationship when the man transferred to long-term care next door. The female ALF resident visited daily and provided oral sex, much to the male resident's delight even though he had a catheter. But his roommate complained about their noise. Once again, there were issues regarding possible health consequences (due to his catheter), as well as privacy concerns. With the assistance of his family, the facility moved him to a private room, but then had to set limits regarding her visits because she began interfering with his medical care. As his dementia with its impaired judgment and impulse control worsened, this resident eventually asked a male nurse to provide sexual stimulation during his care. His focus was purely on his pleasure, and he was losing all sense of propriety. *If your father or mother became involved in a similar scenario, would you intervene? Why? At what point would you intercede? How would you intervene?*

A widowed male resident in his late seventies was bedbound from a stroke. His sexual urges were still operating, and his son personalized his half of the room with posters of scantily dressed, voluptuous young women. This resident would masturbate regularly, much to the dismay of the female aides and residents who could see him *in flagrante,* as the old saying goes. This resident certainly had every right to masturbate, but privacy is a top concern in a facility. The issue here was that he could not move to close his curtain. A remedy was found whereby he would ask the aides to pull his curtain and close the door when he wanted to masturbate. This respected his rights as well as that of others.

With younger nursing home residents, these issues can get even more complicated and delicate. For example, a middle-aged, divorced MS resident became friendly with a new male resident. The residents both were able to give legal consent to sex with one another, but they were not married or in a committed relationship. They requested a room together which was granted, and began sexual relations. This female resident was bedbound because of her MS which meant the aides had to clean her and change the bed after every sexual act, something they felt went beyond their duties. The staff balked at providing this sex-related care, as it was something they were uncomfortable with and certainly had not been trained to do. Additionally, a few months later, the male resident (and erstwhile boyfriend) became interested in another female resident, sparking jealously, hurt feelings, and arguments. *What would you have done in this scenario if you were the nursing home? How much should the aides be required to do? Or, if this involved your lonely and incapacitated mother who wanted a boyfriend, how would you counsel her?*

The Need for Touch

Loneliness and the need for touch will surface in different ways in a nursing home, and it's usually a challenge to the facility as well as the family. This may be as innocent as two widowed residents becoming friendly and holding hands, dining and attending activities together, developing a bond that helps them weather the nursing home chapter of their lives. Sometimes, however, there will be only one interested party, such as the ninety-year-old man who tried to hold hands, kiss, and even fondle a female resident's breast. She did not want any contact, but didn't know how to keep him away. The nursing home intervened on her behalf.

In another situation, a widower would sit every day in the foyer holding hands with two lady friends, one on each side. He was comfortable with this arrangement, often smiling shyly, but the women would often become jealous and bicker. Or, another resident who missed having a man in her life, would attach herself to every new male resident even if he had a wife who visited regularly. One resident with "mild cognitive impairment" seemed to enjoy this woman's attention and said he "didn't want to hurt her feelings by pushing her away." His wife, however, didn't share his noble leanings and protested.

Sometimes a resident's sexual feelings and needs will be directed toward staff. Most often this will involve a male resident who makes sexual comments or propositions a female aide, touching or grabbing her breasts or buttocks. The aide, typically young, does not know how to set appropriate limits and is often worried her job will be at stake if she objects. As a result, the CNA will often smile with nervousness while the male resident takes this as a "go ahead" sign and continues. These sexualized interactions most often happen during care or in the bathroom or shower, since there is closer physical contact between the resident and their aide. And the resident, who may well have at least some dementia, mistakes this as an invitation for intimate behavior. This pattern may be further reinforced if the aide is openly warm, friendly, or caring by nature, confusing the resident as to the true nature of the relationship. There have been situations where the resident has announced that the aide is their boyfriend (or girlfriend), and then wanted their exclusive attention and care. Or, they claimed that the two of them were going to leave the facility and marry, and so forth.

In such instances, the nursing home will intervene and educate the aide as to how to set appropriate limits. Sometimes, however, the solutions are to transfer the aide to another unit, or the CNA only provides care for that resident with another aide present. This is to avoid (unfounded) complaints of sexual abuse, and return the relationship to its rightful balance. But this change may also upset a resident who has been harboring fantasies of a loving and intimate relationship, and now they feel cast aside as if they have lost a loved one and left abandoned in an uncaring world. As human beings we all need to feel connected, valued, and loved. If we lose this basic connection and validation to another, or with a group, it's as if we've lost our moorings in life and do not know how to continue on our own, alone, vulnerable and helpless, the more so if we are old and infirmed.

> The biggest disease today is not leprosy or tuberculosis,
> but rather the feeling of being unwanted.
> ~ Mother Teresa

"Nobody Cares"

A common refrain voiced by nursing home residents is that "no one cares about them," and no one wants them. Certainly not their family if they don't visit enough, because if family members cared, they would "take them home," or so they believe. Not their friends (if they are still alive), who no longer come calling. Not the staff, who are paid to do their caretaking, and no matter how good, reliable or considerate, can never be "family."

As Mother Teresa suggests above, we all want and need to

feel connected to others who want us. It's part and parcel of the human condition since we are all born helpless and dependent on others for our physical survival as well as our emotional sustenance. Consequently, we have a deep seated need to feel we are important to someone, and they will love us enough to care about us and not discard us along the way, especially when we feel vulnerable. This is closely aligned with the feeling most residents have that they've "lost everything in life" once they became too old and too sick to do for themselves and remain independent. They'll often say they have "no future," and with that comes the feeling they have "nothing left to live for" since they can no longer "do" like they used to in their daily living.

When our sense of whom we are and self-sufficiency is undercut, fearful thoughts and emotions surface and swirl around us like a dusty storm that disorients even the most intrepid traveler. It's much different when we were younger and had a "future." That was when we were able to plan and do something to change our life, as well as ease our helplessness and vulnerability. In our elder years, there is no visible future or aspirations, no ability to "do" – something which well may have been the implicit bedrock upon which we built our identity and self-worth.

Although "doing-ness" is the staple of youth and middle age, "being-ness" in the world is something we need to develop and focus on as we grow older. **Beingness** is not geared to trying to control, produce, or achieve some goal now or in the future. When we spend our entire lives focused on doing, achieving, and trying to control life, we come into our senior years unprepared for the fact we can no longer "do" and must now exist as something different, and even unknown. In all probability there will be no future successes, especially significant ones, as our busy doing-ness grinds to a halt. As a result, some residents become preoccupied with what they've failed to achieve in life and now have no opportunity to achieve.

We all know what "doing" is. After all we "do" every single day starting in early childhood, all the while growing stronger in our physical and mental abilities. But if you ask someone what "being" is, they'll usually draw a blank. Yet, deep down we all naturally know beingness, even though it was programmed out of us with the collective drive to survive and its belief that beingness is less valuable, even worthless, and will result in lazy, non-doing self-indulgence. However, beingness and "not doing" are actually two different states, although they may look somewhat alike when viewed superficially.

What is beingness as opposed to doing-ness? Think of the timeless moments when you felt peaceful, content, full, and complete, when you weren't busy doing something "important" to get something "important" so you could feel good about yourself. For example, "being" is gently holding a baby rather than focused on changing diapers, feeding, bathing, or thinking about what needs to be done tomorrow at work. "Being" is sitting in your easy chair and petting your cat's silky fur, the cares of the day long gone, and the mind quiet. Or it's watching the sun silently set in a blaze of color while over your shoulder the moon gracefully rises and the stars come out of hiding. It's not what we "do," but rather it's when *we quietly connect with life's innate wonder and goodness, with the small nourishing pleasures that relax us deeply.* In that instance, we can rest in the timelessness and fullness of the moment: nowhere to go, nothing to do, nothing to think about, nothing to defend, no one to please, nothing to prove.

Old age will challenge all of us to "be" and let go of the busyness of achieving a valuable identity and a future, to rest in the moment and enjoy the simple joys of a human existence, even if it's in a nursing home.

If we don't relearn and develop our innate skill of beingness before we get old, then when we become elderly we are too likely to succumb to feeling lost, unimportant, unwanted, worrying, and yearning to return to the fantasy of a more satisfying time in life.

Such residents cannot feel satisfied and peaceful in the here and now, and with that, sadness and depression creep in, often resulting in the more familiar and toxic symptoms of depression (see below).

In the last chapter on aging well, we'll explore simple ways to support our beingness as well as ward off some of the pitfalls old age and infirmity present. For now, practice your 4 - 4 breathing; it is a readily available gateway to beingness on a daily basis, and it only takes a few moments.

> What you thought before has led to every choice you have made, and this adds up to you at this moment. If you want to change who you are physically, mentally, and spiritually, you will have to change what you think.
> ~ Patrick Gentempo

Depression

According to the National Institute of Mental Health, depression in both men and women age sixty-five and older is a major public health problem. Yet only 10 percent or so receive treatment for depression, and that may only consist of medication prescribed by their primary care physician.

Depression among the elderly often occurs with medical illnesses and disabilities; and will last longer than depression in younger adults. As a result, elder depression is frequently confused with the effects of multiple illnesses and subsequent medications. With long-term care residents who cannot clearly express their experience or symptoms, it's often difficult to delineate what the problem is, its causes, and the best course of treatment. In addition, brain imagery studies in the depressed elderly have shown impaired brain function and size thought to be linked to reduced blood flow through brain blood vessels, as well as decreased neurotransmitters which are important to a sense of well-being.

Although depression falls into several categories based on severity and duration, the most common **symptoms of depression in the elderly** include:

- Sadness or feeling "empty" (but many seniors deny feeling sad and depressed);

- Feelings of guilt, worthlessness, helplessness, being "a burden," having "no future;" tearfulness or crying episodes; feeling unwanted;

- Anxious and worried, often related to an underlying sense of loss or being unable to do or manage customary responsibilities; including financial worries;

- Loss of interest in once pleasurable activities or hobbies;

- Social withdrawal or isolation;

- Fatigue and decreased energy (which also results from illness or surgery); slowed movement; lack of motivation, "What's the use? thinking;

- Sleep difficulties (which can result from pain, medications, etc.);

- Weight or appetite loss;

- Memory problems, difficulty concentrating and making decisions (which may or may not be related to dementia);

- Increased use of alcohol or drugs;

- Neglecting personal hygiene and care;

- Increased physical complaints or aches and pains;

- Thoughts of suicide, suicide attempts, or preoccupation with death and related fears; and a significantly increased suicide rate in elderly white men.

Not every depressed elder will exhibit every symptom, and moreover their symptoms may fluctuate over the course of their senior years, periods of illnesses, and nursing home placement.

There are several groups of **risk factors** that have been found to contribute to elder depression. These factors or stressors include the following:

- **Health problems** such as sudden or chronic illness and disability; chronic or severe pain; damaged body image due to surgery, amputation, or disease; fluctuating and declining mental abilities; decreases in brain activity, blood supply, and neurotransmitters as we age, particularly with certain medical conditions; accumulations of toxins and pollutants, including side effects from medications; poor diets and dehydration; chronic alcoholism and drug use.

- **Isolation and loneliness** resulting from living alone and having few if any friends, co-workers, or other social contacts; decreased ability to make new friends or find new, meaningful activities; physical separation or estrangement from family members; decreased mobility; loss of driving privileges; and limited or no active support system.

- **Loss or reduced sense of identity and purpose in life** due to retirement or loss of work, financial standing, or social status; loss of past roles; physical limitations or inability to do certain activities and manage self-care.

- **Recent losses** such as death of spouse or partner, children, other family members, friends, and pets; relocation or loss of home. Moreover, unresolved grief from previous deaths and losses, such as the death of children, can resurface in later years and lead to a greater sense of aloneness and sadness.

As you can see from this brief summary, depression expresses itself in many different forms, more so the older we get as we confront the multiple stresses of aging. Furthermore, depression reduces a senior's ability to rehabilitate after an acute illness, surgery, or injury. And over time, depression negatively affects everyone's immune functioning, not just seniors.

With a rehab resident it's difficult to separate out whether their depressive symptoms are the result of their illness, surgery, anesthesia, and/or medications (and thus *situational* and will probably resolve on its own or with limited intervention) or whether we are seeing a long standing depressive decline that will interfere with health and recovery, and will require a higher level of treatment.

In long-term care, studies have shown that depression significantly increases the likelihood of death from illnesses. Depression is often underdiagnosed and untreated with up to 35 percent or more of residents experiencing depression of varying severity and duration. In addition, depression exacerbates chronic pain, and chronic pain will trigger depression, and typically both will need to be addressed. So what are the most effective **treatment options**?

For decades, the most effective course of treatment for depression has been "talk therapy" or anti-depressant medications, which must be monitored for side-effects and compatibility with other medications and conditions, or a combination of these treatments.

With elderly nursing home residents, verbal therapies have been found to be less effective since they may be less talkative in general, unwilling to discuss emotions, distrustful of mental health professionals, and worried they will be labelled as "crazy" or "insane." And, if they have moderate to significant cognitive impairment, they may be unable to integrate new information and interventions, as well as develop a working therapeutic relationship.

The issue may come down to whether a fiercely independent, stubborn resident with some cognitive decline is able to change their life long thinking that they must "do" and achieve goals, or, whether they can let go and simply "be" in the moment in the nursing home and find satisfaction in daily commonplace activities. Some can, even quite easily, but some cannot, due to their mental decline and ingrained personality traits. And some refuse to consider the "being" option, even though they are depressed, miserable, and have no ready recourse. *Which one best describes your resident? Which one will you be in your elder years?*

> The aim is to balance the terror of being alive with the wonder of being alive.
> ~ Carlos Castaneda

When a Second Opinion is Warranted

Probably many readers have heard or seen old movie images of ECT or Electro-Convulsive Therapy, and were stunned by the process. ECT involves sending a burst of electricity through the brain; and as a result, is commonly known as "shock treatment." However, ECT is still around, and is considered a treatment of last resort. It is used most commonly for severe depression that does not respond to medications and psychotherapy. Developed in Europe in the late 1930s, it fell into disfavor, and then made a resurgence around the year 2000 after improvements in the process were made. No one knows exactly how ECT works, but it does work well for some patients.

Typically, ECT consists of a series of treatments which must be done in a hospital setting after the patient receives a muscle relaxant and general anesthesia. ECT has been successfully used with those over the age of sixty-five, including age seventy-five and up (termed "old-old" in the professional literature). However, it's important to know that *the health status of the patient becomes more important the older the patient is – meaning there are real concerns if ECT is used on old-old nursing home residents, none of whom are in excellent health or they wouldn't live in a facility.*

In over twenty years of working in many Florida nursing homes across several metropolitan areas, I have never seen or heard of a nursing home resident receiving ECT. A few residents had received ECT many years previous to their nursing home placement, *but none while in a nursing home, and certainly none at an advanced age.* There are side effects with ECT – the more so the older the patient – including memory loss, confusion, and delirium. In addition, the infirmed resident will experience heightened stress and fear due to being transferred out of a facility they know and to a hospital, and then undergo a series of treatments they probably do not understand and find scary. Furthermore, *there are newer anti-depressants that have proved effective with elderly residents and these should always be tried first.*

Given all this, **if you receive a recommendation for ECT for your old-old resident, especially from an Administrator or other personnel who are not physicians who can discuss treatment options, please get a second opinion from a geriatric psychiatrist as well as a full medical evaluation. ECT with an old-old nursing home resident should never be taken lightly.**

> In moments of discouragement, defeat, or even
> despair, there are always certain things to cling to.
> Little things usually: remembered laughter, the face of
> a sleeping child, a tree in the wind — in fact, any
> reminder of something deeply felt or dearly loved. No
> man is so poor as not to have many of these small
> candles. When they are lighted, darkness goes away
> — and a touch of wonder remains.
> ~ Tombstone inscription in Britain

The Past is the Present

Miss Bertha inched her wheel-chair closer to the nurse's station. She was a quiet woman, dignified and well liked. She often read her Bible and seldom said a word in the nursing home.

Miss Bertha had been born before World War I, in another America most do not remember, and few care to think about. She was born a poor sharecropper's daughter in the Deep South. Once she grew up, she never married or had children.

The Nurse Manager and I were talking when out of the corner of my eye, I saw Miss Berta drop something white that looked like a tissue or a hankie. Without even thinking, I bent down, picked it up and handed it back to Miss Bertha. Miss Bertha became agitated, her thin body shaking.

I glanced at the nurse who knew Berta well. She shrugged her surprise, her eyes wide.

"What's wrong Miss Berta? Shall I throw it away?" I asked.

"White people aren't supposed to do that," she finally said, tears in her eyes.

"They should have," I replied softly. "We're all 'God's children,' whether we know it or not."

Hearing these words, Miss Bertha calmed down, while the nurse and I fell into a pit of sorrow for what gentle Miss Bertha must have endured in her life that she never deserved.

In nursing homes, you'll meet people from all walks of life from every corner of America who have experienced the gamut of human experiences, from the highest high to the lowest low. Some, like Miss Bertha, are so old they grew up in the shadow of slavery and the pervasive hatred of anyone different or unknown. They were battered by segregation and poverty, the Great Depression, and the horrors of two World Wars. They were shaped by these larger forces as well as their personal experiences, and for some residents, these memories are never far from their consciousness. Before we judge and reject a bad-tempered, prejudiced, and even demented resident who has lost respect or consideration for others, it's best to remember what Atticus Finch told Scout in *To Kill a Mockingbird*. "You never really understand a person until you consider things from his point of view...until you climb into his skin and walk around in it."

With some residents, I've had to discuss how the world has changed in their lifetimes, and how as a result, their beliefs, attitudes, and responses also have to change — at least to some extent. For example, it's not uncommon for residents to call minority aides by derogatory racial or ethnic slurs. This is especially common behavior in white residents who feel they've lost control over their lives and want to lash back at the ones who are apparently running their lives. One tiny woman who was born around 1900 routinely called the aides "n******," oblivious to the staff's reaction or that this hostility might recoil against her when she needed their assistance. I spoke to her about her language, and she explained, "I grew up on my granddaddy's planation in Kentucky. I was used to ordering them about, not them talking back or ordering me."

We discussed the issue further, as I explained to her that she was now living in an institution with well over two hundred different individuals or more (counting residents, staff, and visitors). As a result, she could not continue to live with, and exhibit, old prejudices, closed-mindedness, and hostility without blowback of some kind. At this stage of life, no resident can afford this; their health requires more care than they realize. With this in mind, together we figured out how she could make peace living in an environment she could not control. Ultimately, she was able to internalize a simple principle, and that is, she was entitled to think as she pleased, but she was not entitled to utter hurtful or hateful epithets. And if she had any complaints against the aides, then she was to bring them to the attention of the managers so they could intervene rather than her trying to balance the scales of power with racial slurs.

Such discussions with the residents often go beyond racial prejudices to include: expanded women's roles, gay rights and marriage, different religions, the Internet and social media, recreational drugs, the younger generation, and immigrants from countries they didn't know existed. Why is this type of therapeutic discussion important? Imagine a resident has an aide from another country who speaks with a heavy accent and there is no option to change aide assignments. Now the resident must learn to work with someone whom they never would have associated with on their own. Or, their daughter divorces after thirty years of marriage to go live with her lover, something unheard of in the resident's church. Or, their granddaughter becomes involved with drugs or announces she's transgender, and so forth.

One conservative Christian resident became upset after her beloved grandson told her he was gay and was going to marry his partner, something she'd believed was sinful. She loved him and wanted to continue their relationship, but since childhood she'd believed homosexuality was "the Devil's work" and that she should stay away from "those people." She also felt she could not discuss the situation with her pastor since his views were ironclad.

Using her religious beliefs, I suggested she look at the situation in a slightly different way since she believed God was the ultimate judge and punisher of our sins. I said, "Why not leave the issue of your grandson's 'sin' of homosexuality and gay marriage in God's hands to do as God sees fit, whether now, on 'Judgment Day,' or in 'the afterlife?' You do not have to assume that role, and this way you could continue loving your grandson without condemning or trying to change him." This reframing – using the resident's own religious beliefs – freed her to continue her relationship with him and enjoy his weekly visits.

These social or life changes will be quite stressful for an elderly resident who must learn how to relate to another person in a new way by somehow reframing or casting aside deep-rooted beliefs. For some old-old residents, our changing world is overwhelming and even threatening – certainly not the America they knew and depended on. Then again, if former President Carter who was born in 1924 in rural Georgia and once supported school segregation, can have an expanded world view, then we all can at any age.

> We become not a melting pot but a beautiful mosaic.
> Different people, different beliefs,
> Different yearnings, different hopes, different dreams.
> ~ Jimmy Carter

Family Challenges

Home-based caregiving to an infirmed senior often becomes a 24/7 job with constant stress and little if any time off. This taxes every caregiver and family, sometimes to the breaking point. Once the infirmed senior goes into long-term care, the stress of daily care and supervision significantly decreases, but new challenges emerge.

Spouses and adult children are usually ill prepared for the enormous change that is happening to their loved one, as well as having to learn to deal with imperfect institutional care, managing ongoing medical care, and later, end-of-life issues. The first step – and the most important – is for the family to truly understand and accept the changes in their loved one, be they physical, mental, emotional, social, or even their overall personality. This is more pronounced when dementia is a primary issue, but it will touch every resident and spouse, adult children, and other closely related relatives and friends.

For immediate family members, a resident's long-term nursing home placement may well mean a drastic change in roles and ways of relating to the resident. For a **spouse**, this entails the loss of a partner in life, that special someone they've shared their daily life with for many decades. Even in a troubled marriage, the couple depended on one another for a variety of small and large activities and responsibilities. Now that support and partnership may completely vanish, with no one ready for this type of sudden and calamitous life change. These elderly wives and husbands will need to learn how to be a supportive spouse in the context of a nursing home, while at the same time build and maintain a life alone, something they haven't done in decades or perhaps never if they married young.

The spouse, partner or significant other will experience many different losses and challenges, including but not limited to the following issues:

- Loss of closeness, affection, friendship, and love, including sexual contact. The spouse may go through a period of mourning for their wife or husband and the life they had together.

- The spouse may feel all alone in life, especially if they have no children or they live far away from where the resident is placed, or do not have an active support system already in place.

- The frequency and quality of conversation with their loved one in general may become limited, reinforcing the sense of loss and being alone. Discussions of how to handle problems may become virtually non-existent, depending on the resident's infirmity and cognitive decline. As a result, the spouse comes to realize they can no longer depend on their husband or wife for any kind of support or assistance.

- For a wife, she may need to quickly learn how to take care of finances and household maintenance after a lifetime of deferring those tasks to her husband. She may not know how to write checks or balance a checkbook. She may not realize what bills need to be paid, where important documents are kept, or control the husband's spending while in a facility if he orders online or via cell phone. She may not drive or know how to get around with public transportation (if needed). She may have followed her husband's lead on many family issues while she exclusively focused on taking care of the home and children, and now all the decision-making is on her shoulders. Women who fit this profile are particularly prone to financial fraud if they do not have someone reliable to help them manage money and finances.

- For a husband, he may have to take on "traditional" responsibilities that were his wife's, and these might include his learning how to cook, shop, clean, do laundry, and maintain the household, including any pets. In some families, the wife took care of finances after the husband handed over his paycheck. If so, then he will need to learn how to take over that responsibility. He will also face the challenge of maintaining social contacts he may have previously left up to his wife. As a result, his new life can quickly become lonely.

- A spouse often feels responsible for their resident's well-being, and so may spend many hours with them in the nursing home. This may be done out of love, but it can also reflect they are lonely, have nothing else to do, and benefit from the nursing home and its staff now becoming their new home base. They may also feel guilty, as if they must "fix" or somehow better their spouse's life and health. At times, they may become overly fussy or hover over their resident or even interfere with care. *Please understand this is part of how they express their love and concern in an upsetting and threatening situation that is out of their control.*

- The spouse or partner may need to handle nursing home finances and medical decisions, which are often more complicated and emotionally upsetting than they realize or acknowledge. It's helpful if a responsible adult child or younger sibling steps in to help, especially if the elderly spouse is also experiencing cognitive decline.

- The spouse may experience a maelstrom of emotions such as: anxiety and worry; fear; irritability and anger; helplessness; hopelessness; guilt and second-guessing themselves for past or current choices; dwelling on the past; "Why me?' thinking; difficulty with memory, concentration, and making decisions; and fatigue. Health problems they neglected during the caregiving period may also surface or worsen, and the spouse may develop or finally admit to depression.

> There are only four kinds of people in the world.
> Those who have been caregivers.
> Those who are currently caregivers.
> Those who will be caregivers.
> And those who will need caregivers.
> ~ Roslyn Carter et. al.

The **adult children** may experience some or all of the following issues, more so if they are the care manager for the resident and have to deal with their parent(s) and the nursing home regularly.

- The mortality and/or impermanence of their parent's life rushes to the forefront of their minds once their parent becomes incapacitated enough to need a nursing home. The loss is no longer a theoretical possibility in the distant future, but a reality in the here and now. This shocks many, who felt as if their parents would continue almost indefinitely, and would not face death and dying for many years.

A parent's decline and long-term placement also brings to mind the real possibility of the adult child's own health decline. Many adult children begin to worry or fear they'll end up like their mother or father – incapacitated; "losing their minds" to dementia; wearing diapers; and/or dependent on strangers in a nursing home for our most basic needs. Their own death suddenly becomes a given.

Moreover, at some point, they have to face their parent's actual death, and all the issues and decisions that come with that eventuality. Few are ready for that unavoidable loss, even if they have had a conflicted relationship with one or both of their parents.

- Another dynamic develops when the adult child becomes a quasi-parent to their mother or father as they take over their care, the management of their finances, and the role of primary contact with the nursing home. This is an unexpected and unplanned role reversal. Some residents resent this, surprised and even angry their children are running their lives and feeling entitled to do so, even to the point of making decisions without consulting them. Others are relieved they no longer have to take care of everything and have someone to lean on who makes life easier.

On the other hand, some adult children – especially those

younger than fifty – continue to relate to their parents as if they themselves are much younger and still emotionally dependent on their parents. But now their parent is a long-term care resident and cannot be that emotional support – upsetting to the unprepared adult child who hasn't yet come to terms with their parent's decline and what nursing home placement means.

- Sometimes adult children continue to bring their problems to Mom or Dad (especially Mom). They will vent and discuss their family issues and problems regularly without realizing their parent is no longer capable of handling this psychological burden. Consequently, some residents, primarily women, will fret, agonize, and ruminate about their children's problems to the point of tears, overwhelmed by the fact they cannot help or even comprehend the problem or available options. The resident still feels responsible in some way, even guilty they cannot help out. At times, when these residents speak about their children and their problems, it's as if they are talking about youngsters, not middle-aged men and women.

Although it's important to include your resident in your life, that has to be balanced with what the resident can deal with and what will not stress or burden them. The residents are physically, emotionally and mentally different and weaker at this stage of their lives, meaning that adult children need to modify and adapt their relationship in light of these new conditions, and be selective in what they share and discuss with their parents.

- Another common challenge is the re-emergence of old hurts, disappointments, and resentments, possibly stimulated and highlighted by the fact that time is running out to resolve them. Parenting and raising a family is often "messy business," with no clear-cut road map to avoid hurts, conflicts, letdowns, and please everyone all the time.

One way this dynamic appears is a desire on the adult children's part for the resident to change and become a different, better person or parent, thereby alleviating the adult children's stress, guilt, and burden. We saw this previously in the Rehab section with the example of Lucy and Marie: Lucy wanted her mother to be understanding and considerate, characteristics that were never prominent in her mother and highly unlikely to surface now that she was in a home.

People usually will not change significantly in their elder years, and certainly not because we want them to, or think they should. For example, if a resident has been stubborn, self-centered, demanding, or critical most of their lives, chances are they will continue to exhibit these traits in some way unless severe dementia or another illness softens their rough edges. Also, keep in mind that chronic pain and illness can trigger negative reactions such as irritability, nervousness, neediness, withdrawal, and constant complaining in someone never known to do so. Be aware that a major illness, surgery, or injury will generally not bring out the best facets of our personalities, at least not initially.

Another family dynamic that surfaces and can cause havoc is old sibling rivalries. For example, the adult children will disagree or argue over their parent's care and medical decision-making. One sibling may refuse to accept the situation, and then pushes the parent or other siblings to do more or even fight against nursing home placement despite the fact they are not willing or able to become the 24/7 caregiver. In the same vein, some adult children quarrel over the resident's belongings and money, even distrusting the sibling who is handling the finances or balking at spending money on behalf of the resident.

Every now and then one sibling will actively intervene to coerce the parent to give them Power of Attorney and move them out of the facility without notice to other family members or the facility. This is done so they can assume financial control or use their parent's money for their own purposes. In more than a few instances, an adult child has used a resident's Social Security or Long-term Care Insurance payments for themselves and refused to pay the nursing home as State law requires. To preserve the well-being of a resident, some facilities have even gone as far as to quietly assumed a large loss and not told the resident of the situation.

The nursing home as well as a psychologist will not get involved in financial disputes among siblings. If elder fraud is suspected, the facility will report it to State officials, who may or may not be able to intervene successfully.

The nursing home experience is stressful for all concerned, and there are no easy answers or shortcuts when this assortment of challenges confronts us. Sometimes the family as well as the resident would benefit from professional help to place these issues in perspective and resolve old hurts and resentments. For spouses and adult children, resolution may not involve the resident at all if they are incapacitated by illness and cognitive decline or dementia. The key is to *first accept the reality of the situation and who they are now, and then figure out what, if any, options are available. Throughout these trials and tribulations, they also need to learn how to take care and nourish themselves.*

As the old adage goes, "If you're going through hell, keep going." So let's take another step and keep moving forward. This is the only way to deal with chronic illness, long-term care as well as life in general.

> Compassion literally means to feel with, to suffer with. Everyone is capable of compassion, and yet everyone tends to avoid it because it's uncomfortable. And the avoidance produces psychic numbing - resistance to experiencing our pain for the world and other beings. Compassion is not being afraid of the suffering in the world or in oneself.
> ~ Joanna Macy

Compassion

When we encounter the suffering of loved ones, especially in a hospital or nursing home, we may feel a strong impulse to turn away and leave, their suffering unpleasant or even frightening. Or, we may want to relieve their suffering, but we don't know how or where to begin. To protect ourselves and not feel the pain of their suffering, we often close our hearts as well as our minds.

As a result, we may resort to criticizing, pushing or exhorting our resident to do more and get better somehow – or else we try to ignore both their pain and our own. In so doing, we close the door to compassion, kindness, and gentleness. To bring it back, all we need to do is ask ourselves, "What can we do in this moment to help another human being during their time of great need? What can we do to brighten their day or ease their suffering a little?

Compassion rests on the basic understanding that *being human involves imperfection, limitations, mistakes, ignorance, not knowing what to do at many moments during our lives, and of course, failures.* It's not our responsibility to take away someone's suffering or life challenges; that's their job or responsibility. It is, however, our job to be kind and gentle to those who are in pain and suffering.

In this world of ours, no one is perfect or infallible. No one is eternally young, healthy, and independent. No one is all-knowing. We all suffer in one way or another, at one time or another – and we could all use a measure of genuine compassion and understanding.

Self-compassion means *applying this same perspective toward ourselves, and accepting we are imperfect, make mistakes, don't know what to do some or most of the time, and suffer like everyone else.* And, we all compare ourselves to others and our learned standards, then disapprove of ourselves and push ourselves to do more, acquire more, and be stronger, smarter, and more perfect somehow. *But in hard times, it's important to be gentle and kind with ourselves, as well as with one another.*

Please don't confuse *self-compassion* with *self-esteem*, which is based on an evaluation where we are "better" than another. Nor should we confuse self-compassion with self-pity, self-centeredness, laziness, or excuse-making. It is none of those things. Self-compassion simply means we accept ourselves, and in so doing, we are kinder and gentler with ourselves.

To bring forth self-compassion, we simply need to open ourselves to its healing simplicity. During difficult periods, we can promote self-compassion by asking ourselves one question: **"How can I comfort myself and ease my suffering in this moment?"**

The answer will not be something big, costly, or dramatic. Certainly it will not be self-indulgent. It will not come or be at the expense of your family or resident. In fact, you'll find it's likely to be small and commonplace. For example, take a day off from visiting; go for a walk in a park or a bike ride; listen to soothing music; attend a yoga or tai chi class; get a massage or an ice cream cone; see an afternoon movie; visit a bookstore; and so forth. It will be an individual answer, of course, unique to each person in their unique situation. Nevertheless, it will help you successfully cope with the stress of your loved one's infirmity and long-term nursing home placement.

Self-compassion will also help you cope with "caregiver burnout" which will likely happen more than once and appear without warning. When you're burned out, you will feel tired, as if you have nothing left, can't stand to see another drop of human suffering, and don't know if you can carry on any further. In the last chapter on aging well, we'll discuss other ways to care for yourself as you face aging in its many forms. But for now, take a little time to practice self-compassion and slow, conscious breathing.

For easy to use exercises and practices to cultivate self-compassion, see Kristin Neff's book, *Self-Compassion* in the Resources section. Also, consider Nick Ortner's *The Tapping Solution*, another easy to learn and effective destressing technique.

> It is not how much you do, but how much love you put in the doing.
> ~ Mother Theresa

Time-Tested Tips

- If you or your loved one has fallen into the dark pit of depression, *please seek professional help*. There are many options available. You need not suffer alone or in silence.

- Ease your stress with self-compassion where you first recognize your own humanity and limitations as well as your own suffering in the situation. Then do something, however small, to nourish and comfort yourself.

- Practice 4 - 4 Breathing to foster moments of relaxation and beingness.

    Breathe in slowly and gently to a count of 4. Imagine your breath going down to your belly button. Then purse your lips and exhale gently for a count of 4. Imagine your breath flowing softly outward, relaxing mind and body, gracefully carrying you into beingness. Repeat three times in a row.

> *Compassion toward others is really a gift for ourselves, because it nourishes us with benevolent feelings and allows us to feel more secure by recognizing our inherent interconnectedness. With the equanimity of an open heart, the slings and arrows of our difficult and frustrating lives find less purchase, and suffering becomes a doorway into love.*
> ~ Kristin Neff

Chapter 9
The Alzheimer's & Dementia Quagmire

"Where did they go?" my uncle asked me, referring to his older brother with vascular dementia and his wife with Alzheimer's disease.

Both were seated near us, busy watching an old movie on television.

"I don't know. Nobody knows." I answered as I glanced at my father and aunt-in-law, neither able to tell us what was happening on the screen. "Parts of the brain die, and with that they go somewhere we can't follow."

My uncle looked back at me, sorrow carving deeper into his once handsome face, the years of caring for his wife exacting their toll – many tolls, unfortunately.

Earlier that week he'd realized his wife had taken another deeper step into the Alzheimer's quagmire. Most mornings he would go to the nearby supermarket at seven sharp so he could be back home well before she woke up. But this week when he returned, she was at the front door in her nightgown, frantically looking up and down the street, and wailed when she saw him, "I thought you had gone and left me."

"I'll have to take her to the store with me. She doesn't like that – it upsets her – but I can't leave her alone again," my uncle had said. Then he told me how he first knew her flighty forgetfulness was something much worse. He'd left to drop off his car at a close-by repair shop, and she was to follow a few minutes later to pick him up in her car. This had been the usual routine over the years when one of their cars needed service. This time, however, she didn't show for over two hours because she had lost her way. When she arrived, harried and confused, she couldn't tell him where she had been or how she finally found the shop. Probably because that incident scared her, she soon thereafter gave her car to her grandson, delighted to help him with his commute to college.

Scenes like these become routine in any family where one of the dementias – including the most common, Alzheimer's – has come for an extended stay. At first, family members dismiss what they see their loved one do, unable to distinguish what is a minor lapse in memory from the beginnings of progressive brain deterioration. But sooner or later the realization dawns that something is wrong, and it's not a passing mistake or the garden-variety changes of an aging mind. This acknowledgement becomes a moment of fear, and then sadness. We've all heard too much in the news, and from neighbors and friends, not to know what this means in the life of our loved one. We may not understand what dementia is or its stages, but we know it as a modern-day scourge that permanently changes lives and the families of the loved one.

As neurologist and best-selling author Dr. David Perlmutter bluntly states, "Alzheimer's is a disease for which there is no effective treatment whatsoever. To be clear, there is no pharmaceutical agent, no magic pill that a doctor can prescribe that will have any significant effect on the progressive downhill course of this disease."

This does not mean that the resident is doomed to a meaningless life as an empty-headed object of pity, derision, or fear. There is much more to a human being than remembering the details of their life, being able to balance a checkbook, or find their way to the grocery store. However, a dementia diagnosis does mean we need to understand a loved one's brain disease so we can relate to them more effectively: With love and compassion, and not fear or anger. In so doing, we also learn how to manage our own stress and emotions, including grief over the losses dementia brings into our lives.

Below is a concise summary of what we currently know about **dementia,** so that we gain a better understanding of what dementia is, as well as the difference between dementia and normal cognitive aging. Moreover, I'll explore the issues dementia presents in long-term care, including the top three mistakes family members make.

Note: Throughout this book the term *dementia* is used more frequently than *Alzheimer's disease*. This is because *dementia* is the global term indicating significant deterioration of mental abilities, and includes Alzheimer's disease among the other dementias.

For more detailed information on the dementias, consult the internet as well as the Resources section where you will find a list of books on dementia from a variety of viewpoints. Two books well worth reading are *Thoughtful Dementia Care: Understanding the Dementia Experience* by nurse Jennifer Ghent-Fuller and *Surviving Alzheimer's* by Paula Spencer Scott. Please know much has been written during the last ten years about dementia and Alzheimer's from the perspective of a caregiver, as well as from clinicians and researchers.

You'll find the available dementia information will vary depending on the year and country of publication, as well as the training, profession, or role of the writer or organization. Any differences you'll encounter in symptoms, diagnostic labels, staging or levels, are usually insignificant. However, what we know continues to evolve as research continues, and subsequent changes in diagnostic criteria and labels are expected. Information about the dementias has changed significantly throughout the last twenty years, and research continues to move forward to find the causes as well as successful treatments. That said, we need not wait for some magic pill in a distant future; we can actually do something practical and beneficial in the here and now. According to Dr. Perlmutter, "The bottom line is…we need to expand the public awareness that modifiable lifestyle factors have a profound role to play in determining who will or won't get this disease."

Finally, if you read any research data, remember that research regarding the "elderly" denotes men and women age sixty-five and up, and "old-old" means either seventy-five or eighty-five and up (usually the latter). Elder research does *not* distinguish between younger seniors and those in their eighties, nineties, and beyond who have different bodies, cognition or mental abilities, psychology and early conditioning, needs, and may respond differently to illnesses, traumas, treatments and medications.

As you read the overview that follows, *keep in mind that every individual with dementia or Alzheimer's disease is unique, and so their symptoms, downward course or progression, and timeline will vary, sometimes significantly. Any concerns regarding your loved one should always be discussed with a physician or neurologist, since dementia diagnosing cannot and should not be done based on information from a book or website.*

> To know how to grow old is the master work of
> wisdom and one of the most difficult chapters in the
> great art of living.
> ~ Ram Dass

"Are they crazy or what?"

A new, petite resident looked up at me from her wheel-chair, her Jersey accent adding a little spice to her speech, her brow furrowed over intense brown eyes. "They shouldn't be here if they gonna act like that."

"Where should they be?" I responded, although I already knew her answer to this often spoken question.

Some residents do not like to be near residents with dementia and want them banished from the facility. Other residents tolerate them easily even if they display behaviors no one likes or can understand. There's no way to tell who will fall into which camp, or whether time will soften a new resident's fear and negative opinion.

"Don't know…but somewhere with others like them," she said, shrugging her thin shoulders.

"There is no other place," I explained. "All nursing homes have residents with dementia or Alzheimer's, and some have the disease more than others and do things we don't like."

She harrumphed and wheeled off to Bingo. I hadn't offered the answer she wanted to hear.

In decades past, to say someone was *demented* meant they were "crazy" or "insane," and should be locked up as far away as possible from the rest of us. More recently, *demented* simply means a person is suffering from one of the dementias. They are not crazy or insane, despite strange or unusual behaviors and/or speech they may exhibit, especially in the later stages of the disease.

Researchers do not know what causes dementia, except those dementias related to a significant (head) injury or illness, a rare genetic abnormality, or chronic alcoholism and other substance abuse. What we are learning is that lifestyle factors play a substantial role as we'll see later in this chapter.

Dementia is a global term for a constellation of symptoms in which memory, thinking, attention, decision-making, judgment, problem-solving, language, social, and perceptual abilities are impaired enough to interfere with daily functioning. Simply put, regardless of the specific diagnosis, dementia symptoms expose *a progressive and degenerative brain disease where parts of the brain are damaged or dying and do not work properly*. For example, imaging studies of Alzheimer's have shown a decrease in nerve cell activity as well as other abnormalities, while in other dementias there might be lesions (dead areas) in the brain or reduced blood supply.

Dementia is not a reflection of personality, character weakness, willfulness or stubbornness, paranoia or mental illness per se. Nor is it confined to any one particular group of individuals. **Progressive dementia** *begins slowly and gradually worsens over a period of years, interfering more and more with daily functioning, including taking care of themselves and relating to others. Symptoms will vary, not only from one individual to the next, but throughout the course of their disease, and even within a single day.*

When confronted by dementia, family members are often confused and alarmed because they do not understand the changes they see in their loved one. To highlight the fact that dementia reflects a degenerative brain disease beyond the individual's control, I sometimes liken the "demented brain" to a "toaster with a short circuit" (an analogy the older generation seems to understand).

As anyone who has dealt with a fickle, shorting appliance will report, it can be maddening to figure out what's happening or what to do to make it work right. One morning the toaster makes perfect toast, just like always. That is, the demented person carries on a conversation where they know who is who, what happened, and so forth, and you think they're back to their normal self. The next day the toaster doesn't work no matter how many times you try it or how much you want toast. This is similar to the demented resident who looks at you blankly when you mention a family member who just left or what they had for lunch ten minutes ago. Then another morning the toaster works, but burns the bread. In this instance, the demented resident becomes argumentative or paranoid for no apparent reason, even contrary to their lifelong way of being. Unfortunately, there is no way to know when the toaster will work and when it will not, or how it will function at any given moment. Over time, the toaster will have less and less "good days" where it toasts bread the same old way, and more and more "bad days" until eventually it stops working all together. **So it is with a demented brain: sometimes the neural connections work, and sometimes they don't, and there is nothing we can do to change it.**

We can also use a computer analogy, something more fitting for a younger, computer savvy generation. The problem with dementia is not with a computer's software programs or an app. Rather, the problem lies in the hardware, specifically, the "motherboard" or "logic board" that runs a computer. If there is a glitch in the motherboard, at first it might only show sporadically, disrupting a program, crashing or locking up when you're surfing the internet or writing an email. It passes quickly, or you reboot or restart the computer and the problem goes away – until the next time. Over time the problem becomes more frequent and widespread, affecting more of the computer's functioning until the system totally "crashes" or doesn't work well enough to do the tasks at hand.

When dealing with a malfunctioning computer, we get frustrated and may fantasize throwing the computer out the window, but we can always get it fixed or buy a new one. Not so with our loved one's demented brain: It cannot be fixed. In addition, we won't understand what is happening; why they can't do the simplest task; why they say the strangest things or repeat the same question a dozen times; why we can't reason with them; why they're uncaring and oblivious to everyone else; or why sometimes they're here and sometimes they're not. We'll feel helpless because we cannot improve the situation. We'll get angry more than once or twice, and have to learn to "go with the flow" and "take it one day at time" when that's the last thing we want to do. This is the difficult, unavoidable state of affairs when dealing with our loved one's progressive dementia.

Whether we like it or not, we need to understand and accept the fundamental reality of dementia in order to move

forward. Getting stuck in anger or despair will not do anyone any good. Much like a small child, the demented individual will not understand your anger or criticism, yet they will respond in some way to the felt disapproval and rejection. In addition, they will not comprehend your despair or worry, nor will they show any appreciation and gratitude for all you do for them. Your efforts simply "do not compute."

> No matter what the relationship was between the parent and child — whatever it was — This [dementia] is going to be extremely challenging because it is not logical. There's no way to deal with it rationally or directly. You don't reason it out. What I've said to so many people is: we always must lead with our love.
> ~ Stephen Hoag

Depending on the **classification** system, there are either seven or eight dementias that are incurable and will worsen over time. The most prevalent is Alzheimer's disease which affects one out nine adults age sixty-five and older. Within people aged eighty-five and above, the number goes up to one out of three adults. According to the Alzheimer's Association, approximately 5.2 million adults have Alzheimer's in 2015, and that number is expected to rise to 7.1 million by 2025 and 13 million by 2050.

Two thirds of the people with Alzheimer's disease as of this writing are women. The latest estimates say that at age sixty-five, women have an estimated one in six chance of developing Alzheimer's while men have a one in eleven chance. There is no available data explaining why women are more at risk. Researchers also say that the disease may begin twenty years or more before the diagnosis, and women may worsen quicker. This underscores the need for everyone, especially women, to address the modifiable lifestyle factors as soon as possible.

Alzheimer's accounts for at least 60 percent of dementia cases, and probably much more. When we include the estimates for all the other progressive dementias, it becomes clear that dementia affects a sizeable percentage of older adults, and by extension their families, society, and the healthcare system. It's also important to realize the majority will remain at home since only a small percentage will be admitted into a nursing home or assisted living facility.

After Alzheimer's, the second most common dementia is **Lewy body dementia** which affects approximately 15 percent of diagnosed individuals, and can result in difficult to manage behaviors and movement disorders. **Vascular dementia** represents about 10 percent of diagnosed patients and is caused by reduced blood supply in the brain. Furthermore, an individual can have more than one of the dementias, further complicating the symptom picture. Moreover, these estimates as well as what we know about the dementias is in a state of flux as new research data becomes available.

A Dementia Diagnosis, and the Stages

Diagnosing dementia is often a knotty and inexact process, and if you read various diagnostic systems or information sources, you will notice there are some inconsistencies and overlap. As a result, **dementia is often diagnosed by its clinical presentation or what the person shows in terms of mental (cognitive), behavioral, and personality changes that affect daily functioning**.

While dementia and Alzheimer's symptoms will vary among individuals, **at least two of the following basic mental functions must be impaired** for a diagnosis to be made.

- *Memory loss; difficulty forming new memories; and, disorientation and getting lost while driving or even walking.* Memory is essential for many daily activities, so when memory lapses become losses and then pervasive deficits, the individual will exhibit increasing difficulties in even the most commonplace daily tasks.

Memory loss proceeds backwards from the present. This means the person will retain distant memories while forgetting recent events and memories – something that makes new learning difficult.

Before you worry that your loved is getting Alzheimer's, please know that memory problems alone do not signify dementia or Alzheimer's. Many older adults experience memory lapses and loss, and these can result from many different causes.

- *Language declines, including impaired ability to read, write, speak, and understand the speech of others.* As a result, communication with others becomes compromised and in the later stages, nonexistent. Individuals who speak English as a second language may lose this ability and revert to their primary language as their dementia progresses.

- *Impaired ability to focus and pay attention; impaired multi-tasking (doing two or more tasks at the same time such as talking on the phone while writing down instructions or directions); and impaired coordination and motor functions.*

- *Impaired higher or executive intellectual functions*, including the inability to: plan; organize information; solve new problems and make decisions; do money math; and, the inability to engage in abstract thinking, everyday reasoning, and common sense judgment. As a result, the ability to perform a sequence of complex behaviors such as driving, cooking, paying bills, managing medical conditions and medications, or adapt to new situations, becomes difficult and prone to mistakes. In particular, processing speed and learning new information becomes greatly compromised. Due to these impairments the individual with dementia is susceptible to financial scams and frauds, and may exhibit an obsession with sweepstakes.

- *Mood and personality changes*, such as irritability or becoming stubborn or angry when frustrated, tired, or told what to do; withdrawal or loss of interest in activities or socializing; being self-absorbed and insensitive to others, including close family members. Other possibilities include inappropriate or impulsive behaviors; paranoia or suspiciousness; anxiety and agitation; delusions (false beliefs that go contrary to any evidence, accompanied by an insistence they are true), and hallucinations (seeing or hearing things that others do not).

Years back dementia was described in terms of seven stages, and even sub-stages within the seven stages. This has given way to a simpler classification of stages or levels: **Mild, Moderate, and Late stages**. Prior to the first stage is **Mild Cognitive Impairment** (MCI). With MCI, the individual exhibits noticeable memory and thinking problems beyond those expected with normal cognitive aging (see below). Sometimes the person is aware they are not thinking "right" or that something has gone awry they can't control. In response, depression, anxiety, and apathy may surface. Usually these changes are not severe enough to significantly interfere with daily responsibilities and activities, especially if they have a supportive spouse or family. Some people with MCI may not get worse for many years, while others develop dementia or Alzheimer's over time. There is no way to determine who will or will not develop dementia.

In the **mild stage** the individual is still functioning independently, but there are more memory and concentration lapses. They may begin having trouble performing work tasks or planning and organizing information. Some individuals are adept at covering up their mental lapses with lots of words, and others believe they are doing better than they are and dismiss any problem or contrary information. At some point, performing complex tasks becomes an ongoing problem and mistakes are more commonplace. Sooner or later they'll need to retire from work, hobbies, sports, and other similar complex activities.

The **moderate stage** is typically the longest stage; and the latter half is often when placement in assisted living or long-term care occurs.

During this stage, the person's cognitive abilities continue to decline and interfere with daily tasks. For example, forgetting to pay bills or overpaying; managing money, loans and credit cards incorrectly; falling prey to fraud and scams; burning food or setting the kitchen on fire; getting lost while driving or having car accidents; difficulty with bathing, laundry or maintaining a clean home. They will become more forgetful, missing doctor's appointments, taking too much or too little medications, or unable to provide their address or phone number. They may confuse words or have difficulty understanding what they read or are told; exhibit sleep pattern disruptions or day-night reversal; or begin having trouble controlling their bladder and bowels.

They may exhibit personality changes such as increased anger and irritability; paranoia or suspiciousness (accusing spouses of infidelity or other hurts); agitation and anxiety; become aggressive; or ruminate on worries yet unable to do anything to resolve them. These worries may be present or past, and either important or relatively minor. The anxieties may involve confusing past and present details or forgetting new details. For example, one nursing home resident ruminated about her daughter's breast cancer, as she could not remember her daughter had recently successfully completed treatment and was cancer free.

In the **moderate-to-late stage**, the dementia patient may wander or attempt to leave the house or facility again and again with little if any safety awareness. They might hoard or rummage through belongings; pace or do other abnormal behaviors such as wring their hands, fold or tear tissues or clothes; exhibit "disinhibition" such as undressing or spitting in public, making sexual comments or using racial slurs without any awareness how it affects others. They may display other impulsive behaviors (again, with little if any awareness of possible consequences). Some may exhibit delusional false beliefs and hallucinations, which can be difficult to manage without professional assistance. As dementia progresses, the individual loses their sense of humor and may become anxious and agitated when teased or told a joke. This is because they no

---

The man in the mirror

A long-term resident complained he couldn't use his bathroom because his roommate was always there. The staff couldn't understand it because his roommate's habits hadn't changed. When I asked the resident to tell me more, he got up, walked to the bathroom door, and pointed to the man, saying, "See, see."

The door had a full length mirror on it and he was looking at his own reflection. He could no longer recognize himself so it had to be the roommate. This sometimes happens in the later stages of dementia. The mirror was removed and the problem solved.

longer can understand jokes, puns, and other word play.

They may also exhibit "sundowner's," wherein their symptoms worsen in the late afternoon or early evening. It's thought low sunlight and impaired vision disorient the individual, or there's a disruption in their internal body clock. The change in symptoms could also be related to a drop in blood sugar: The individual needs to eat, but will not be able to ask for food to tell anyone how they're feeling, assuming they can tell they are hungry.

Once those afflicted begin to forget the basic details of their own personal history – where and when they were born; who their parents or siblings are; and significant life events – they are showing signs of decline into **late-stage dementia.**

In **late stage** dementia or Alzheimer's, the person may not recognize other people, including close family members. They will not fully understand what is told to them, and may speak in incomplete or incoherent sentences, or utter random words unconnected to what is happening around them. Some exhibit severe agitation, depression or a flat expression. Some become fixated on ideas or past events; or pinch, swat away or hit caregivers because their behavior is perceived as a threat. At this point they need twenty-four-hour care, and may exhibit significant impairment in sitting, standing, walking, and swallowing. They are also increasingly prone to infections.

At the end of the disease, the resident may be curled up in a fetal position or move around the bed erratically, unresponsive to others or outside stimuli until they finally stop eating and drinking altogether as they prepare for death.

As you can see from these brief descriptions, dementia and Alzheimer's follows a progressive, downward course where the individual's neurocognitive symptoms worsen and they are less and less able to function in the world. Family and friends will often say, "They are not the same person," and they are not, but let's not lose sight of their humanity, their inner presence that makes them unique. They are simply someone with a brain disease, and as worthy of our love, kindness, respect, and compassion as anyone else with or without a major, debilitating illness.

> I am saddened when I hear these words – this is not the person I knew – because those words objectify the person suffering from Alzheimer's. When you objectify a person you also dehumanize them. Once dehumanized the person becomes a villain.
> ~ Bob DeMarco

Normal Cognitive Aging

As we age, our brains will change along with the rest of our bodies. Consequently, every one of us will experience cognitive aging (not to be confused with a disease like Alzheimer's or dementia). How much change, or what type of change occurs, varies greatly from person to person, and may shift from one day to the next.

According to the Institute of Medicine (IOM), cognitive aging is a natural part of aging, with the changes variable and gradual. Unless an older adult has a chronic illness or disease, the older brain shows only minimal neuron death, even if overall neuronal function declines. As a result, during our elder years we can still learn and enhance our wisdom and expertise. Furthermore, seniors report less negative emotions that younger adults, as well as a greater sense of satisfaction in life.

We can take steps to support our cognitive health and better adapt to the natural changes we'll experience. The most important action steps to take are:

- Be physically active on a regular basis;
- Reduce cardiovascular risk factors such as high blood pressure, high cholesterol, diabetes, and smoking;

- Regularly review mediations with your physician to avoid negative cognitive effects;

- Be socially and intellectually engaged in life; and continue to learn and exercise your brain with cognitively stimulating activity (music, reading, puzzles, etc.); and

- Get adequate and refreshing sleep. (If you have sleep problems, consult a professional.)

It's also important to remember most seniors live independently, and our personalities remain fairly stable throughout their lives. Not everyone is destined to develop dementia or live in assisted living or a nursing home, although many will need rehab services at some point. We all experience age-related physical changes that will affect our lifestyle to some extent. These include hearing and vision impairment, as well as changes in smell, taste, and touch and temperature sensitivity. There is also the increasing probability of arthritis, hypertension, heart disease, diabetes, and osteoporosis, among other ailments.

Psychological research has shown the speed with which we process information slows as we age. As a result, we probably learn new information more slowly, and require more repetition and demonstration. As older adults will attest, there also will be memory lapses, the so-called "senior moment." This especially true for long-term memory, as short-term memory shows less age-related decline.

We also lose some of our ability to divide our attention and multi-task, i.e., do two or more tasks at the same time. And, although we'll probably experience more difficulty finding words, our wisdom, learning, and creativity can continue until the end of our lives.

In a nutshell, we need to accept, support, and adjust to our cognitive and physical aging, as well as manage change and stress effectively. There is no need to be pessimistic and give up living a satisfying and meaningful life. Sure, our life will be different, but we just have to adjust and modify our old ways of doing things. Chances are strong we may even learn some new ways. Life is always changing; that is its nature, and we must change with it.

> The secret of health and happiness lies in successful adjustment to the ever-changing conditions on this globe; the penalties for failure in this great process of adaptation are disease and unhappiness.
> ~ Hans Seyle

Stress Management

Change is a natural part of life, and that includes changes that come with increasing age, cognitive and health decline. **Stress** occurs when we need to adjust to changes in our environment and life circumstances. We either adapt or resist the changes – and that resistance is what leads to greater stress and negatives effects.

So, we can either use the energy of stress as a call to action to move forward in life, or we can resist and suffer the inevitable consequences. The choice is ours, and it will occur over and over again during the course of our lives.

Some stress related changes are fairly mild, while others are significant and life-changing such as the illness or death of a loved one. In addition, we each have a personal pecking order of stress, as well as how we respond to stress. For example, retirement for one person could be a boon, while for another it's a shocking loss of who they are and what they do in life, and they tumble into depression and illness. One person may react to rush hour traffic with road rage, while the driver in the next lane sings along with the radio and waves merging cars in front of them.

Decades of research have clearly shown that stress affects our physical, mental and emotional health, although often slowly and without our awareness. There are many effective and seemingly small and inconsequential steps we can take daily to relieve stress, but they must be done on an ongoing basis. A little here, a little there while we lead stressed lives and blindly follow old habits or "new" impaired thinking does not work. In the Resources section of the Appendix, you'll find numerous suggestions for stress management techniques; check your favorite bookstore or online for other possibilities. An easy and effective technique that can be done anywhere is the 4 - 4 Breathing, introduced in Chapter 1.

Seniors with mild-to-moderate cognitive declines will experience heightened stress if they have difficulty remembering important details, figuring out priorities, and solving problems, especially those related to money, health, and medications. They will be hesitant to discuss their difficulties or ask for help, often fearing criticism that they are "stupid," defective, or gullible (especially if they've given money and assets away). This ongoing stress then triggers more troubles, taxing their already burdened physical and psychological health in an unforgiving downward cycle. When this happens, it's a cry for help, and hopefully a responsible and caring family member can step into the picture to help. If the elder goes into a facility of some kind, this usually takes the pressure off and they soon show improvement, assuming they accept their new placement.

> Sixty feels exactly like fifty, with aching feet and more forgetfulness.... but your inside person doesn't age. Your inside person is soul, is heart, in the eternal now, the ageless, the old, the young, all the ages you've ever been.
> ~ Anne Lamott

Dementia & Long-term Care: Top Mistakes

Not every nursing home resident has dementia, but most will at least have some cognitive and memory impairment as they age and suffer various illnesses. This will naturally interfere with their adjustment to long-term care, relationships with others, cooperation with care, and general well-being.

Most facilities are practiced with dementia since they deal with it regularly, but this does not mean they handle every situation or behavior perfectly. Dementia is a challenge to everyone regardless of whether the resident is quiet and compliant, depressed, agitated, argumentative, paranoid or aggressive. It's important never to treat the resident as an object, defective or worthless, or meet their anger and aggressiveness in kind. Till their last breath, they are a human being worthy of our understanding and compassionate care.

This written, there are a host of common mistakes that family members make as their loved ones go through dementia and its changes.

- **Mistake #1: A Failure to Accept**

In long-term care, the primary mistake families make is not accepting their resident's dementia and its downward progression. Some family members adamantly deny their resident has dementia, dismissing their lapses as "senior moments;" overlooking the problems they had at home and what brought their loved one into a facility; and/or disregarding the changes that have occurred over the course of their placement. In these instances, family will actively disagree and even argue with medical staff, implying or outright accusing staff of over-diagnosing, incompetence, or that they and the facility have some ulterior motive for diagnosing dementia.

Some families seem to think staff derives some kind of pleasure or satisfaction with a dementia diagnosis or that their resident will be treated more poorly or discarded somehow as a result. More than a few family members have repeatedly refused to agree to medications that could enhance their resident's well-being, and minimize the importance of their significant mood and behavior problems. They often say they don't want their loved one sedated or sleepy, even when it comes to a resident suffering significant pain who cannot get relief otherwise. On the other hand, a few families demand certain medications against medical advice, saying their information (gleaned from the Internet, or from someone who may or may not know the resident) is superior, or that they know their resident best.

For example, an eighty-six-year-old woman was exhibiting more serious cognitive declines, quickly becoming lost and confused whenever she came out of her room. She would become anxious and agitated, could not be calmed down for hours, and refused meals, care, medications, and her usual activities. At times she hurried to the front door and tried to leave the facility. Yet her son refused to accept she was suffering from dementia as well as the recommendation that she would benefit from transferring to the closed dementia unit. In his mind, she was just a little confused and forgetful. After all, he "had lunch with her every week," and they "carried on a conversation;" to what extent, he could not tell us. Nor did he know what she did or did not remember.

I suggested a Mental Status Exam of the resident with her son and daughter-in-law present so the son could get a better understanding of his mother's condition. He agreed, and we proceeded. His mother could not answer any item correctly. Once the resident left us, with a smile still on her face, I asked her son how he thought his mother did. He told me he thought she did "fine." I then showed him her test answers, all of which were failures, and explained the scoring to him. He was shocked. It was only then that we could have a discussion of the difficulties she was experiencing in the large, open unit she resided in, and why a closed dementia unit would be more helpful. His mother was soon transferred, and she quickly adjusted, calming down with no exit-seeking, once again accepting meals and care, and even joining in activities she had refused for months. This woman's inner life became less chaotic and stressful once she was in a smaller, closed unit that could offer her more support.

Another long-term resident came into the facility with some degree of moderate dementia, and slowly declined into an aggressive later stage. He'd often see things that weren't here, speak in disorganized and incoherent phrases, fail to understand what was said to him, grab the aides inappropriately, or go limp when they tried to change his diapers. He was a big man, and when he began swatting, kicking, and punching the aides, the situation became serious and unsafe. His wife refused the doctor's recommendation for medication, saying she didn't want him sedated, and that he wasn't demented and could converse with her "rationally" (something the staff had not seen in over a year, as he could not respond to even the most basic mental status questions at this time). His wife would proceed to talk about his past professional accomplishments, as if what he did thirty or forty years ago had any bearing on the present or his brain disease. She also refused to have a neurologist evaluate her spouse, even though she apparently did not trust or believe his attending physician.

This situation continued for months until the Administrator gave the wife an ultimatum: either comply with the doctor's recommendation or transfer him to another facility. The wife finally agreed, medication was prescribed, and the resident quickly calmed down.

One variation of this aforementioned scenario is when the wife is significantly younger (by twenty to thirty years) than her husband and cannot accept his dementia or his decline. Here, she cannot process that she is quickly losing him and the life they led. So she will dismiss diagnoses and treatment recommendations, insisting on her idea of what's best and will keep him "young" and alive.

Another fairly common scenario is an older husband who cannot accept the fact his wife, whom he has depended upon emotionally, is demented and failing. He will regularly browbeat her so she capitulates to his superior reasoning, all in the name of motivating her to "do more" and return to a higher level of functioning than she is capable of.

These types of spouses are often difficult and demanding because they will not accept the medical staff's diagnoses or recommendations, much less enter into a meaningful discussion regarding their spouse's dementia and age-related decline. Typically, they will even refuse anti-depressants or similar medications for their resident – no matter how depressed, weepy or agitated they become – saying they don't want them sedated or "dopey."

In my nursing home experience, psychotropic medications are *not* over-prescribed, nor are residents heavily sedated zombies. I did see this happen in the 1990s, but not lately. Sometimes, medications are necessary for the safety and well-being of the resident, *as well as that of others who could be hurt by their dementia fueled actions*. In the situation above with the aggressive resident, he should have been on medications for months; that would have prevented many incidents as well as the increased stress on everyone. But if the family does not accept a dementia diagnosis, it is impossible to have a thoughtful discussion regarding options when such problems arise.

If your family as a whole distrusts the care being provided or treatment recommendations, or believes the facility or healthcare professionals are incompetent or have ulterior motives for a dementia diagnosis, seriously consider transferring your loved one to another facility. If this seems too drastic step, seek an evaluation with an independent specialist, such as a neurologist or neuropsychiatrist, for dementia issues. One way or the other, family must establish trust in the present facility or transfer their demented loved one.

- **Mistake #2: The Expectation of Normalcy**

The second most common mistake is related to the first: If family refuses to accept the resident's dementia or their subsequent decline, they will continue to expect the resident to be their "normal" self. Consequently, they will try to reason with them (the most frequent tactic), and expect the dementia resident to exert superhuman will power to change their mood and behavior. When their reasoning doesn't work – and it won't – the family member often gets angry and critical, further complicating the situation.

What families do not understand is **that reasoning is a higher mental function that is one of the first to go – forever**. Dementia requires us to understand and relate to the individual differently, and expecting them to somehow overcome a diseased brain **does not work**.

My primary recommendation to family members is to educate themselves regarding dementia and Alzheimer's, and what to expect from the disease process.

Second, I suggest they develop a positive working partnership with the nursing home staff, including the various medical providers. Realize that dementia progresses downwardly, and it will change how your resident thinks and behaves, as well as what they need at any particular moment. Their dementia will follow an unpredictable course, and you will need to learn to follow it, for it cannot be dictated.

Last but not least, take care of yourself. This will be a slow, challenging marathon. And throughout it, keep asking yourself, "What is best for the resident?" A helpful approach to answering this question is to make a comprehensive list of pros and cons that take into account their dementia symptoms. Review it often to ensure you are up to date and they are being served by every decision.

> Worrying about what will decline next or wishing you could recapture something from the past will only prevent you from being in the present moment. Even as flawed and difficult as it may be, that's where life is.
> ~ Carlos Gibbons

• Mistake #3: The Belief You Need to Solve Every Problem

As every caregiver will agree, dementia presents many challenges, often "at the drop of a hat," and always when you least expect it. Nursing homes are obligated to notify family members of any incident, or significant developments, with their residents.

But this notification does not mean you, as the responsible family member, need to *solve* the problem. Sometimes the issues are unsolvable, or require other remedies you cannot provide, but can be supported in one way or another.

And at times, absolutely nothing at all needs to be done by you.

For example, years ago a ninety-three-year-old dementia resident would wander the halls and occasionally return to his old room, which was now in the AIDS unit. One day he entered his old room and saw a urinal with yellow liquid on a bedside table. He quickly drank it (probably thinking it was juice), then left to continue his stroll. When a family member found out about this (a young nurse had seen what happened and informed her), she became very upset, and quite concerned her loved one would develop AIDS. When the seasoned Director of Nursing heard of this, she told her not to worry because at his age, he would die before any symptoms developed. And sure enough, this elderly resident died peacefully a year later at ninety-four, never having developed AIDS or even HIV+ status.

So, when you receive news of a new development, the first step is to remember to take a few deep, calming breaths. Remind yourself about the nature of dementia and nursing home life.

Then, ask yourself, "How important or critical is this behavior or problem? Do I really need to do something right now, or let it go? Is it up to me to resolve the situation?"

Sometimes you need to accept that unfixable problems will arise and surrender control, so neither you or your loved one becomes unduly stressed. This way, you can be more present and supportive of your loved one, as well as experience your own peace amid the passing storms.

> I had the good fortune of being around a number of Alzheimer's patients in the last three years of my mother's life. She was in a care facility that was devoted to just people with memory-loss issues. I found those people engaging and generous in ways that I had not imagined.
> ~ James Rebhorn

"Personality Changes" Caused by Dementia

In her book *Surviving Alzheimer's*, Paula Spencer Scott describes four broad categories of "personality changes" caused by dementia. I have not seen any research on these patterns, but my clinical experience agrees with these basic groupings. Sometimes these personality changes are an extension or exaggeration of the resident's original personality, but sometimes they are not, or are even contrary to their lifelong personality.

Keep in mind these are not clear-cut categories since they may overlap or change over time. Nevertheless, they can be useful to better understand the changes families see in their loved one. The four most common categories, with my additions, are listed below.

1. *Depressed and/or anxious, worried, or at times agitated with no discernible trigger anyone else can identify or remedy.*

   The resident may have had a history of depression, tragedy or trauma, but sometimes none the family can recall. Some people, however, hide their inner distress and turmoil so well that others do not recognize it. It's well known depression negatively affects our immune functioning, hastens cognitive decline, and results in persistent unhappiness and dissatisfaction with life. Depression that is moderate to severe, and is not short-term or situational, should be evaluated by a healthcare professional, including the need for anti-depressants.

2. *Apathetic and unmotivated to the point the resident refuses to get out of bed, has no interest or motivation to do anything, even once enjoyed activities.*

   Their affect or facial expression is often flat and unemotional. They show no initiative except to say "No" in one way or another, even if they have agreed to get up, or attend an activity or outing. Basically, no one is going to motivate or move these residents.

3. *Paranoid, suspicious, frightened, angry, and hostile which can result in accusations, hallucinations, false beliefs, resistance to care to the point of lashing out and becoming aggressive.*

   When the seven stages of dementia classification were used, these behaviors were usually seen when the resident's dementia was progressing from the later stages of moderate dementia (stage five) to the late stage (stage six). Once these residents' dementia deteriorated into the late stage, these behaviors would either cease or decrease in frequency and intensity. These residents are the most difficult to manage, and their negative behaviors usually result from both brain changes and situational or environmental factors. They need to feel secure in a predictable and non-threatening environment. At times, placement in a closed dementia unit will need to be considered.

4. *Passive, contented, without a care in the world, and in the moment.*

    These residents are the easiest to manage. They usually adapt quickly to the nursing home if it is supportive and stable (e.g., not chaotic, or providing poor or rough care that threatens them). Typically, they say very little, so family members and aides need to be observant to pick up hints that they are uncomfortable with something in their environment; they don't feel well or have pain; or their hearing or vision are worsening. Moreover, their demeanor may look childlike (described below in the "eternal now of dementia").

> People think it's a terrible tragedy when somebody has Alzheimer's. But in my mother's case, it's different. My mother has been unhappy all her life. For the first time in her life, she's happy.
> ~ Amy Tan

The "Eternal Now" of Dementia

For some residents, dementia is like a new friend who takes them away from bad and painful memories and into the quiet comfort of the present moment. Old traumas and tragedies no longer haunt them, old fears and obligations subside, and the need to please and be approved of fades away. This can take various forms, yet with all the individuals experiencing it, there is a peacefulness and acceptance of life that silently shines forth.

If you spend enough time with such individuals, you'll find your mind going quiet, and with that comes a sense that all is right in this eternal moment. Nothing to do, nothing to say or think about, nothing to prove, and nowhere you have to go. This state of beingness or "no-mind" is what mystics have alluded to, and what modern meditators seek; although without the negative effects of brain deterioration.

Somehow dementia can bring the meditative "eternal now" into the life of some residents. Some smile sweetly and "go with the flow," comfortable in their new home. Others sit quietly and share their love through warm, liquid eyes. And in that loving moment, there is a lesson for all of us.

One eighty-three-year-old who was sexually abused as a child finally felt safe enough to tell someone what happened, and find relief from the shame she had carried privately for decades. This woman also hoarded small towels, which initially upset the staff even though it calmed her anxiety and gave her control over something in life. Because of the useful purpose these towels served, I recommended to the Director of Nursing that this resident be given the eight daily towels she desired, and afterwards her conflicts with the staff diminished. Then, as her dementia progressed, her painful preoccupation with the past receded more and more until she forgot the father who abused her, and found lasting peace.

Another resident, a combat veteran with a long history of nightmares, finally slept through the night with the aid of his dementia, while others forgot their personal horrors of war, internment, or losing homes, families, and children. For these individuals, dementia is a gift like no other.

> Be still. It takes no effort to be still; it is utterly simple.
> When your mind is still, you have no name, you have
> no past, you have no relationships, you have no
> country, you have no spiritual attainment, you have no
> lack of spiritual attainment. There is just the presence
> of beingness with itself.
> ~ Ganagji

"Are We Doomed to Get Alzheimer's?"

No. The biggest risk factor for developing dementia is advancing age, something we cannot control. However, lifestyle factors also play a key role in whether or not someone develops a degenerative brain disorder such as Alzheimer's. This is great news, yet also poses a challenge to change our ways – the sooner, the better.

There are risk factors for dementia and Alzheimer's we can do something about right now, today. These risk factors include: heavy alcohol use; atherosclerosis (buildup of fats, etc. in artery walls, reducing blood flow to the brain); cholesterol; hypertension or high blood pressure; depression; diabetes; high estrogen levels; high homocysteine blood levels; obesity; and smoking. All of these are considered "modifiable lifestyle factors" we can improve, beginning today.

Alzheimer's research has also identified genes which result in a much greater risk for developing early onset dementia (which is relatively rare). The research also says that a family history of dementia puts us at greater risk for dementia. However, many people with a family history or genetic predisposition never develop dementia, and many people without a family history do. Research continues in order to better understand the dementias, as well as genetic factors and how we can influence their expression. Until then, we all need to take steps to lead healthier lives.

A person's health isn't generally a reflection of genes, but how their environment is influencing them. Genes are the direct cause of less than 1 percent of diseases: 99 percent is how we respond to the world.
~ Bruce Lipton

Time-Tested Tips

- Get to know dementia and/or Alzheimer's. Gather information as well as become familiar with your loved one's dementia experience. Every person with dementia is unique, and their symptoms will fluctuate and change throughout the rest of their life. Their dementia, however, does not mean we cannot relate to them even though it will be a different relationship. For practical wisdom and suggestions, read *Surviving Alzheimer's* or visit *www.TeepaSnow.com*.

- Do not fear normal cognitive aging. Lead a healthy lifestyle, and enjoy life.

- What has dementia taught you? How has it changed your understanding or appreciation of life?

- Have you taken the time to nourish yourself and cultivate self-compassion? This is vitally important if you are dealing with a family member with dementia, whether at home or in a facility.

- Are you practicing conscious breathing to slow down the advancing march of daily stress? Consider taking a few slow, calming breaths prior to entering a facility, your loved one's room, or whenever you begin feeling stressed, tense, angry or emotional. It will make a difference.

GETTING OLDER BEING HERE

Wherever you are, be there totally. If you find your here and now intolerable and it makes you unhappy, you have three options: remove yourself from the situation, change it, or accept it totally. If you want to take responsibility for your life, you must choose one of those three options, and you must choose now. Then accept the consequences.
~ Eckhart Tolle

Chapter 10
Healing in Dying

"I want to die." Josephine looked straight into my eyes, her jaw set, telling me without words she was serious and unyielding.

I was with her because the attending physician had requested a consult: Josephine was refusing her medications and would not discuss her refusal with any of the medical staff. The staff didn't think she was suicidal, but they and her family were concerned and didn't know what to do.

"Why did you stop taking your medications? What's the problem?" I asked.

I already knew the problem could be almost anything: medication side effects; a nurse or aide the resident doesn't like; a roommate that's getting on their nerves; lousy food they're tired of eating; a family dispute they want settled; unresolved grief or depression with a wish to die; or something new no one's ever heard before.

"I've made up my mind. No one is going to change my decision," Josephine said. "I have the right to refuse."

"Yes you do, and I'm not here to change you. I just want to know what's happening that you made that choice. It's not a common decision residents make." (This is true: Only a small minority of residents make a clear-cut decision to stop treatment that will result in a relatively quick death.)

"I'm very sick and I know, my heart doctor told me. I don't want to live like this."

Josephine was indeed an extremely sick woman, but with no reported significant depression or dementia. The nursing staff said her daily life and care were becoming increasingly difficult and painful as she weakened and couldn't do much for herself.

"Are you in pain? Feeling bad some way?" I asked.

"Yes, and I don't want to be kept alive to please the doctors or my children. I'm eighty-six and I'm ready to go," Josephine said. "It should be about what I want, not other people."

"Yes, it is your decision, and I respect that. How can we help make your remaining days better and less painful?"

Josephine looked back at me and tilted her head. "No one's asked me that. They just want me to take pills and do therapy. My kids don't want me to die, but I tell them, we all do."

"So, let's talk about how we can make this better for you. It that all right?" I asked.

She nodded in response.

As you have just read, I did not try to talk Josephine into doing the medically correct thing or please others by taking medications that were prolonging her life. She was in pain, clear in her position, and had the legal right to make her medical decisions, which includes the right to refuse treatments. A power struggle would have served no purpose except to isolate Josephine at a time when she needed our understanding, respect, and support.

My first goal when consulting with a resident is to forge an alliance with them, so I can get more information about the problem they're facing and search together for solutions. With Josephine, we discussed how she felt, and what she wanted and didn't want. Then I spoke to the Director of Nursing (DON), and brokered a solution whereby Josephine accepted two medications that would help her live each day a little more easily while she waited for death's embrace. The DON took care of matters with the staff and doctors to ensure no one tried to force her to change her mind.

The last piece of the puzzle fell into place quickly once her family knew about Josephine's choice and how she wanted to live the remainder of her life.

Josephine died peacefully two weeks later.

> You don't get to choose how you're going to die, or when.
> You can only decide how you're going to live.
> ~ Joan Baez

Prolonging Life or Prolonging Death

In every nursing home, death is always waiting in the wings since the residents are elderly (age sixty-five and up) and very sick. Despite this obvious fact, we see residents and families expressing attitudes similar to those in our modern society – namely the fear and refusal of death.

Like most Americans, new residents, regardless of their age and health, try to avoid seeing or thinking about death, even denying our mortality is a natural part of their lives. It is not unusual for residents and/or their families to refuse or postpone discussing or drawing up Advanced Directives (legal documents indicating preferences regarding end-of-life care). This attitude – that death is somehow a failure rather than an inescapable feature of all life – is reinforced by several social influences.

First, we are living longer than ever before. As of this writing, the average U.S. life expectancy for men is seventy-six years, while for women it's eighty years. When greater longevity is coupled with our youth-oriented culture and advertising, even elders believe they are not going to die until they are ready, and then it will be in their sleep. Consequently, they do not feel the need to face their own mortality or address end-of-life preferences with Advanced Directives, a Living Will or a DNR (Do Not Resuscitate Order on cessation of heartbeat). In addition, for some elders and their families, religious beliefs play a significant role if those beliefs require that life must be prolonged at all costs.

Second, medical science and technology have made great strides in the last few decades. As a result, Americans have also come to believe we can be youthful, active, and independent, and live virtually forever. And if we do develop a health problem, we believe it will be resolved quickly with the latest pill or high tech procedure, rather than make lifestyle changes that require effort and discipline.

For decades the medical mindset has been to prolong life, often shelving quality of life considerations as if they are inconsequential or detrimental to the extension of life. Some expect the surge of aging Baby Boomers to challenge these attitudes as costs and quality of life issues become more pressing concerns, but it will take a determined effort to overcome entrenched attitudes as well as the underlying fear of death.

Based on reports from residents, their families, and my own personal experience, it appears doctors do not know how to clearly inform and discuss the probability that a loved one is facing death. To the extent doctors do talk about death, they often offer medical information that is vague or even contradictory. The difficulty here might be medicine's inability to accurately predict death until it is imminent. These troubled waters are further roiled by the fact that most people do not feel comfortable asking a doctor to be more specific, or whether their condition is terminal and the success of treatment low or painful.

For example, in my experience with my father's cancer, I had to specifically ask the doctor if my father's condition would kill him soon, and the only focus should be on pain management. Another time with another close relative, I had to ask the attending physician whether he was saying if an infection was treated it would prolong life as well as pain. Only then did I receive clear answers that could guide my decision-making, in accordance with my loved one's wishes.

It struck me the doctors were uncomfortable telling me the truth, as if they didn't want to cause me pain or hurt my feelings.

However, what I needed was clear information and fearless guidance so I could understand the medical reality. I wanted this information as I could put my own distress, confusion, and grief aside for the moment; I would deal with that afterwards.

Residents and family members who expect and sometimes demand every medical intervention available – without taking into account the increased pain, discomfort, and helplessness or decreased quality of daily life that could result – complicate the process of dying even further. This insistence for more medical care is often due to their denial of the reality of their loved one's health status; differences of opinion among family members; fear and denial of death in general; and an inability to let go of a parent or loved one for fear of feeling alone in life.

There is also the specter of guilt when a family member feels as if they should have tried harder, persisted longer, or somehow done more for their loved one. And if they had done any of that, then their loved one's decline and death would have been avoided, and no one would have to deal with death and what it means.

Some adult children feel they should give back the care parents gave them, with increased guilt if the parent is a constant complainer who is never satisfied. They behave as if their job as their children is to please their parents and make them happy, even though this is a job no child regardless of age can fulfill. Accordingly, they ask, insist, and demand more and more medical treatment, never stopping to consider the results of each decision or asking their parent (or other loved one) what they want in the last chapter of their life.

Here are a few examples to highlight these issues and choices. A sixty-five-year-old rehab resident returned from seeing her oncologist brimming with excitement, saying she would begin "a new round of chemo as soon as she completed rehab." Unfortunately, that was not what the oncologist wrote to the nursing home. The "progress note" said there would be no more chemotherapy because the resident's body was failing and she was expected to die soon. The medical student who had accompanied the resident at her appointment privately asked the oncologist why he didn't tell the patient the truth about her test results. The oncologist answered he could not bear to tell her she was dying.

The nursing home now faced a dilemma: neither the medical staff, nurses, nor social workers could tell her the grim news because it was the oncologist's responsibility. Yet having no other recourse, the facility asked me to tell her since I had a good rapport with her. I was hesitant because it is not the job of a psychologist to provide medical updates. (Psychologists are mainly available to patients after the medical news is given, to help the residents.) In the end, I agreed since no one else seemed available, and the woman would have several important decisions necessary to make in the coming days. Despite the resident's initial shock and many sad moments that followed, she was able to die in peace, surrounded by her loving family.

Here are some questions to ponder if death is near, and you or a loved one are facing extremely difficult choices about suggested medical choices and treatments, end-of life- care preferences, and so on.

- If this was you or your loved one, what would you want? Be specific.

- What questions would you ask the doctor?

- Would you ask about the test results if the doctor didn't mention them?

- Or, would you take the situation "one day at a time" and push aside any thought of death until you had no other choice?

- Would you take the time to figure out your preferences for end-of-life care and document them before it becomes a necessity?

Another resident, newly admitted into rehab, complained she had surgery and was placed on a feeding tube without her permission. I asked if she had Advanced Directives or a Living Will, and she answered, "No."

I said, "What usually happens is a senior did give permission and doesn't remember (not unusual under the circumstances), or their next of kin gave permission because they were unable to, or they came into the ER without any documents and unconscious or unable to voice their preferences. The hospital is then obligated to provide all the care that's needed to save their life.

For the future, if this is not the kind of medical treatment you want, put what you want and don't want in writing. And, talk to your family so they know your preference and will carry them out."

Like most residents, she had never thought of spelling out her preferences or telling her family.

> If you judge people, you have no time to love them.
> ~ Mother Teresa

Reasonable Quality of Life

One day, ninety-four-year-old Ellie Mae announced she wanted to stop her thrice-weekly dialysis. The nurses in the facility as well as at the dialysis center tried to talk her out of her decision since it meant certain death, and soon. Ellie Mae would not budge, saying, "Enough is enough." Since she had no family, the nursing home now faced the issue whether Ellie Mae had the mental capacity to make this medical decision.

When I spoke to Ellie Mae, she was clear as to the reasons why she was stopping treatment: dialysis was too uncomfortable, both during and after; she had no quality of life since she was bedbound most of the time; she understood stopping dialysis meant death in about two weeks; and she was "ready to meet [her] maker." After hearing this, I informed the facility that from my perspective, Ellie Mae was competent to make the decision to stop dialysis. Ellie Mae stopped her dialysis and enjoyed almost three weeks of feeling good and attending activities she had given up. Then she fell into a coma and died quietly.

Here is another example. An eighty-six-year-old resident felt a small lump in one of her breasts. Her doctor recommended a mammogram, followed by a biopsy and a mastectomy. The resident agreed to every one of these recommendations, terrified of cancer. This woman died shortly after her last surgery, having spent almost three months in high emotional and physical distress not even thrice-daily anti-anxiety medication lessened.

Since cancer is said to grow much slower in the elderly, the nursing staff wondered if the testing and surgeries had been necessary. "Was this resident, at age eighty-six, served best by this course of treatment?" they asked. Unlike Josephine and Ellie Mae, this resident let her fear of cancer and death rule her decisions, possibly led astray by incomplete medical information and a 'prolong-life-at-all-cost' attitude.

Another nursing home resident had malignant breast cancer for ten years and never gave it a second thought. She refused all treatment and let nature take its course, never feeling pain despite the obvious eroding of her body.

- What would you do in circumstances similar to these women?
- Would you be willing to live with a cancer diagnosis and forego treatment?
- Would you have the courage to stop life-saving treatment and stand your ground when well-meaning medical personnel recommend otherwise?

Consider a different response, for example, in the case of a ninety-three-year-old long-term resident who had chest pains and was immediately sent to the hospital. Tests revealed a failing heart, yet his wife and children insisted on the only treatment that might save him: open heart surgery. He had the surgery, then spent over six weeks in intensive care without improving and in considerable discomfort. Finally, he died.

This or similar stories have been repeated many times over in nursing facilities throughout the country. There are many examples of families being told the resident is facing death, yet demanded more treatment, never thinking of the suffering that could result from additional treatments. Some embark on this course in the belief the doctors and their tests were wrong, and that more could and should be done. Others say "No one told them the diagnosis was terminal," or explained the prognosis; or the doctor did not go into detail regarding the consequences of a procedure or treatment; or they thought that there is always the possibility of a miracle.

In addition, some families report they agreed to their resident receiving a feeding tube because they were told their loved one would die a painful death from starvation and dehydration. (*Not true.*) Then some were shocked to see their resident suffering with indigestion, vomiting, or diarrhea; trying to pull out the tube because it was uncomfortable or scary; and/or not fully recovering as they expected. It's important to keep in mind that long-term care residents will stop eating as their bodies begin to prepare for death, and medical authorities now say this appetite loss is not painful, but is a natural anesthetic that eases death.

When my mother was diagnosed with advanced adrenal cancer and there was no recourse, she begged me to make sure her younger brother (in his seventies) did not make any medical decisions for her. She believed he would agree to any treatment because he could not accept her death. I said yes, and used her preferences to guide my decision-making in her final days. This made it easier for me, since my standard question to myself and the doctors was, "Would the suggested treatment prolong her life *and* her suffering?" When the answer was it would prolong both her suffering and death, the issue became solely how to make her as comfortable as possible; nothing else mattered. As a result, additional treatment did not occur, and I was by her side when she died at peace in a hospice center.

As individuals we do not need to conform to the prevailing attitudes of more treatment no matter what quality of life follows. Yet in the heat of the moment, it is difficult and gut-wrenching to make seemingly life or death decisions for someone you love. I write "seemingly" because the decision is *not* life or death, since the individual is suffering from one or more chronic illnesses or a catastrophic injury, and their condition is terminal. For most people, however, it *feels like* a life or death decision. In reality, however, *it is a decision whether to prolong life with a reasonable quality of life – or prolonging and delaying death at the expense of quality of life and well-being, and possibly causing more pain and suffering.*

If you are the adult child, spouse, and/or care manager for an elder, have you discussed their end-of-life preferences with them? Could you keep your emotions at bay and consider all sides of the medical equation, especially if your loved one did not specify their end-of-life preferences?

Have you thought about your *own* preferences? Have you informed anyone else about them, specifically someone whom you trust? Have you had them written down?

> Those who have the strength and the love to sit with a dying patient in the silence that goes beyond words will know that this moment is neither frightening nor painful, but a peaceful cessation of the functioning of the body.
> ~ Elisabeth Kubler-Ross

Healing in Dying

My years working in nursing and assisted living facilities made me confront death over and over again. I've learned through my own life as well as working with others that when faced with significant illness, loss, tragedy, or trauma, we must find a larger perspective or else we sink into despair, bitterness, anger, resentment, and/or a quiet depression that robs us of our emotional well-being. As a result, I've read many different books on death and dying from every conceivable angle, and tried to remain open to any viewpoint that could shed light on the subject. Being a witness to others dying also prompted me to ask myself what I wanted for *my* end-of-life care. It also made me realize how important it is to die in peace, to be "satisfied with my life" as one resident put it.

What does it mean to be satisfied with one's life? What would that look like?

Certainly it's not having every wish come true or be showered with riches and acclaim; that may come to a few, but not to most of us. Nor does it mean we'll never experience heartache and disappointment; that is a part of every human life. As I've aged, my definition of being satisfied with life has also changed, and actually gotten much simpler and easier to achieve.

I encourage you to ask yourself: If you were at the end of your life, would you be satisfied with your life? If not, what would it take for you to be satisfied with your life? Could you welcome death in peace?

When faced with their approaching death, residents often voice fear about the actual process of dying and whether it would be painful. Once reassured that either hospice or the doctor can manage any pain with medication to ease the dying process, they relax and that worry dissolves.

Others voiced that they did not want to be alone – something that cannot be guaranteed since the moment of death can come at any time. We all die alone as we are born alone, even if we're surrounded by loved ones.

Many of us will try to make final sense of our lives or correct some confusion about life; make peace with estranged loved ones; apologize for thoughtless misdeeds; or make amends for selfishness and past abuse.

And for some, their own beliefs stand in the way of a peaceful death.

For example, one ninety-year-old resident fought against the nurses on her death bed as she tried to get out of bed, saying she, "…didn't want to meet Satan!" This lady was a devout woman who believed we are born sinners and meet Satan once we die, then we fall into the fiery pits of hell for all eternity. In her unwavering religious view, there was no other possibility, no chance of redemption no matter what she did. As a result, she was adamant about fearing and avoiding death – something she could not do. She had to be sedated to avoid injury and to give her some measure of comfort. I often wondered whether her church served her with these beliefs that could never bring her peace of mind and heart, regardless of whether or not she had not been perfect in her life.

When working with someone's religious beliefs, I first ask them to define or describe their beliefs. Often, the problem as well as the solution lies within those same beliefs. And if the resident is agnostic, atheist, or has more of a scientific worldview, I begin at the same place, asking them to tell me more about their beliefs.

Another ninety-year-old resident, Elizabeth, realized she was approaching death and worried she had sinned and would be denied "God's grace" and entry into heaven. She was a religious woman who'd been taught to fear "Judgment Day," but unlike the woman above, her beliefs were open to questioning and fine-tuning. My conversation with Elizabeth about sinning and God's judgment went more or less as follows.

"When we die, we are judged according to our sins, and that determines what happens to us — heaven or hell, yes?" I asked.

Elizabeth nodded that I had accurately understood her belief.

"So, how have you sinned?" I probed.

Elizabeth shrugged her thin shoulders and said nothing, sinking deeper into her wheel-chair.

I'd known Elizabeth for some time and she was well liked in the nursing home, unfailingly kind and understanding of others. I'd met her family and their love for her shone brightly. I couldn't see how she had so badly wronged anyone, but this was her story we were unraveling.

"Well, have you committed some heinous crime like murder, rape, torture, abused children – that kind do thing?"

She shook her head, and still said nothing, which was unlike her.

"So, when you talk about being a sinner, you're talking about the everyday sins all of us commit at some point, like being selfish, unkind, gossiping, or being mean and disrespectful, that kind of behavior? And of course, we should all try to do better and clean up our mistakes, make amends if we need to."

"Yes," Elizabeth mumbled, nodding her head.

"You also said that God is 'all knowing,' meaning God knows everything. And, if God knows everything, then one of the first things God must know is that we're fallible and imperfect down here, yes?"

"Yes," she answered, wrinkling her sparse brow.

"You also said God is 'all merciful' and 'all loving,' yes?"

She mouthed a 'Yes.'

"Let me see if I got this right. God knows we're imperfect human beings. God is 'all merciful' which means God is compassionate and forgiving, even in the face of our imperfection. And God is 'all loving,' meaning there are no conditions to God's love. We don't have to be perfect to receive God's love, right?"

Elizabeth nodded slowly.

"So, if you believe God is all knowing, all merciful, and all loving, what is there to be afraid of at Judgment Day?"

Elizabeth looked at me, still nodding. She seemed a bit confused, and that's a good thing because it meant her black-and-white beliefs were being shaken up. I had repeated her beliefs back to her, but fleshed out or amplified with what they logically meant in everyday life. Because we tend to follow our beliefs uncritically, once we question them, they open up to us to reveal what truth or false ideas lie inside.

"Why don't you think about that, and let me know next week?" I told her, and took my leave.

By the following week, Elizabeth did not feel any inner conflict or fear of dying. Her beliefs about God, sinning, and Judgment Day were now in alignment with what she felt was true within.

> We are all afraid of being alone – of not being accepted, of not being loved, and of not fitting in. We deeply ache to be loved and accepted and the fear of not experiencing these things torments us all. Now here's the crazy secret – just naming this fear, admitting it to another …can become the touchstone for authentic, deep, honest soul communion and fellowship. It can actually become redemptive. It's a miracle.
> ~ Fred Grewe

In the months leading to his death, an eighty-one-year-old resident questioned whether his life had meaning. For the first time he told of the horrific abuses he and his mother suffered at the hands of his alcoholic father. He held a secret belief – quite common to victims of abuse – that he deserved it somehow. He also was bothered by his decision to keep distant from his two sons as they were growing up.

At one point, I asked him if he ever drank to excess, and he said, "Never touched the stuff." Then I asked him if he ever hit his wife, and he said, "No." He explained he loved her, and would never do that to the one person who stood by him for sixty years, and gave him and his children a good home. When I asked him why he chose to remain apart from his sons, he said quietly, "I didn't want to hit them. I still remember what that felt like."

I then explained the cycle of abuse, whereby each generation blindly follows the pattern of violence, abusing children and wives as well as alcohol and drugs, and passing abuse and self-hate down the line. When he first became a father at twenty-three, he'd made a decision that stopped the abuse cycle by choosing to keep some distance from his sons to avoid beating them, and letting his wife discipline them. Although his relationship with his two sons suffered by this distancing, he still had time to make amends and he did by telling them about his childhood and his subsequent choices.

Here was an ordinary man who'd taken a heroic step that changed the likely course of his family pattern. With the knowledge his life had more meaning than he realized, this man died at peace two months later with nothing left unspoken between him and his sons.

> Before death takes away what you are given, give
> away what there is to give.
> ~ Rumi

Healing and transformation is always possible, and it can come in a variety of ways, sometimes in a casual whisper, sometimes profoundly and in an instant. Here's another example of healing that can happen at the end of one's life and have a positive ripple effect, this one from my mother.

Unlike my father who never spoke about emotional matters, my mother was not only interested in psychology, but insightful.

As she neared her death, she thought over her life and shared an important insight with me.

When she divorced my father in the early 1960s, she thought it didn't matter to him because he was emotionally closed and stoic. But as the years went by and she learned more about psychology from *Oprah* and other talk shows, she realized the divorce had also hurt him, only in a different way. I asked her if she'd like me to share this with him, and she said yes. A few days later when I was back home and visited my father at his nursing home, I asked him if he was interested in hearing what she told me. He said yes. I told him, and despite his dementia I could see he took it in and visibly relaxed. He was touched that someone had acknowledged him and the pain and loss he suffered in life.

Regrets of the Dying

Author Bronnie Ware in her book, *The Top Five Regrets of the Dying*, conveys the most common regrets dying individuals reported during her hospice work. I've added some elaboration based on my experience with residents at the end of their life.

I wish I had…

1.…**the courage to live a life true to myself, not the life others expected of me**. When someone is on their death bed, they can sometimes see the choices they made, and that they often followed old, deeply rooted habits instead of their true or authentic self. Unfortunately, when we get old and our health plummets, it is often too late to follow our dreams.

What dreams have you pushed aside or let lie fallow?

What choices have you made that did not support what is true for your inner self?

Did you blindly follow guilt or pleasure-seeking, or did you make a choice?

Some people believe if they are true to their inner dreams, they are selfish and inconsiderate of others or snubbing family obligations. But this is old social conditioning talking with its nonexistent analysis and insight. After all, does fulfilling our dreams always have to be at the expense of our children and loved ones?

For example, let's say a man has harbored a lifelong desire to draw or paint, but pushed that aside to earn a living for his family. Can't he do a little something every week to satisfy that dream? That might involve turning off the TV and spending an hour a week learning to draw from books or the internet, or experimenting with a watercolor kit. He might wait until the children are grown or he has retired before he tries something more involved and costly. In any event, his dream need not be postponed forever and become a regret.

If we look closely at how we spend our time, we can see what choices undermine or nourish our true self.

What are your dreams?

What are your regrets?

What do you need to do so your life is in line with your true self?

Make a list of realistic and easy action steps you can take.

Please ensure, however, that your dreams are realistic and pragmatic, not pie-in-the-sky fantasies. Dreaming and wishing to win a $300-million-dollar lottery is not realistic because you cannot do anything to change the incredibly low odds. And as we all know, money by itself will not bring happiness or a life true to our inner self or free from the expectations of others. On the other hand, dreaming of doing art, completing a family tree, putting in a vegetable garden, or writing a memoir are all doable. With the internet, there is a world of possibilities waiting for us to explore.

If you do nothing yet still hold on to litany of lost dreams, you may well find yourself stuck in the quicksand of regret on your death bed. Dying often takes some time and few die in their sleep without a period of declining health, with plenty of time for mulling over the past and regretting.

We cannot change the past, but we can certainly move forward in life.

What can you do right now, even if it's a small step, to further a dream and nourish yourself?

2. **I wish I had not worked so hard**, and missed my children growing up and I had nurtured greater closeness with a spouse or partner.

This is a sentiment often voiced by the elderly men I meet. The older generation in particular was trained to believe the man should be the breadwinner and the woman should take care of the home and childrearing. The result is often dissatisfied, stressed, closed-hearted men who die fairly young from heart-related ailments without exploring other options and deeper yearnings.

Money and status, the proverbial "keeping up with the Joneses," or pursuing and achieving the "success" images and stories from advertising and other media rarely, if ever, results in a happy, satisfying life.

> Most men lead lives of quiet desperation
> And go to the grave with the song still in them.
> ~ Henry David Thoreau

If relationships and family are important to you, what can you do today to nourish and strengthen those relationships?

Do you take the time to be with your children, or grandchildren, and enjoy life?

Do you talk to your spouse and listen to them so you can grow closer?

Are you expressing the song within you?

3. **I wish I had the courage to express my feelings**.
We all suppress and deny our feelings because that was the way we grew up in order to please others and maintain some semblance of peace. Recent research has clearly shown that repressed emotions and a life spent pleasing others, results in chronic stress; that, in turn negatively affects our health and well-being. (See Chapter 1 for more information on our early programming.)

Bronnie Ware adds, "We cannot control the reactions of others. Although people may initially react when you change the way you are by speaking honestly, in the end it raises the relationship to a whole new and healthier level. Either that or it releases the unhealthy relationship from your life. Either way, you win."

4. **I wish I had stayed in touch with my friends**, and encouraged those friendships instead of succumbing to the busyness of life.

Are there any old friends you lost track of and would like to reconnect with? It's never too late to try, and with the rise of social media like *Facebook*, it can be relatively easy.

Research on cognitive aging and dementia has shown that being socially engaged and having a support system is important to our health. Take a step or two toward becoming more involved with others and intellectually stimulated before it's too late and you're no longer able.

Introverts, who usually make close relationships with only one or two people, often feel uncomfortable reaching out to form new relationships late in life. So for them, the loss of already formed relationships can leave them alone and isolated. Nonetheless, they too can cultivate greater connections with others through attending group activities at an adult learning or senior center, or even through the Internet.

5. **I wish I had let myself be happier.**

We are truly creatures of habit and we fear change with an unhealthy passion, even to our own detriment. This leads us to live lives ruled by old habits, patterns, and unconscious conditioning. Happiness and self-compassion are a choice, and recent Positive Psychology research has demonstrated they can be cultivated.

Ask yourself, *"What am I choosing today? In this moment? Can I allow myself to enjoy the simple pleasures of a human life, and in so doing, sweep away the habit of mental regret-making?"*

> Death is not the greatest loss in life.
> The greatest loss is what dies inside while still alive.
> ~ Tupac Shakur

Nearing Death

Based on her years working with hospice patients, psychotherapist Kathleen Dowling Singh wrote *The Grace of Dying*, which describes what happens as a person nears death. This "nearing death" period can last from several weeks to the last few days as the individual prepares physically and psycho-spiritually for death.

In her work Singh describes the qualities she's observed during this period as the person accepts death and makes peace with their imperfect life. These include the following qualities (with a few additional comments).

- **Relaxation**, or a letting go of the struggle to live, and with that, a surrender to dying.

  Based on what a few residents have said, I often suggest to those facing death that they "relax into the body," and allow this natural process to take them where they need to go. Most are surprised to hear this since it is contrary to our conditioning that tells us we must control life somehow. In short order, however, the resident begins to relax once they realize there is nothing else they can do. It has all been done by this point, and all that is left is the last period prior to death.

- **Withdrawal** from the world and its distractions, and a turning inward.

- **Going within** one's own experience with no interest in others, activities, family disagreements, money, legacy, and so forth.

- **Silence** or reduced communication.

  The resident has little if anything to say, and it takes too much energy anyway. Due to this turning away from the world and others, the individual may appear depressed. This is not "depression," but another step away from this world and toward death. They don't need anti-depressants or similar medications, although they may need comfort measures as well as compassionate loved ones and staff. If we sit with them for a time in this silence, we can feel the subtle quality of stillness and beingness emerging. This is also a good time for gentle 4 - 4 breathing.

- **Brightness or light** that shines from the eyes and skin.

  One resident in her early seventies struggled to accept her terminal diagnosis, but she finally did, and was also able to reconcile with her estranged daughter. Two days before her death, I walked into her room to say "goodbye," and saw her half of the room filled with bright light. In that moment I knew my friend would transition peacefully and without difficulty. I silently thanked her for coming into my life and sharing this gift of light.

- **Openness** to the sacred, and a focus on love.

  For the dying resident, the past with all its mistakes, disappointments, regrets, and missed opportunities is a fading memory that doesn't need to be mulled over or discussed any longer. What was, was, and it is not present in this moment; and when that happens, all that is left is love.

- **A knowing** or a greater, unspeakable understanding begins to unfold.

  The resident may be able to make sense of their lives and the nature of life and love to a larger or deeper degree, and even share some of that knowing with us.

- **Experience of perfection**, or a subtle, yet unmistakable sense that everything is okay as it is.

  Nothing to do, nothing to say, nothing to be, nothing to change – and in that, there is peace and freedom.

> It is not the end of the physical body that should worry us. Rather, our concern must be to live while we're alive. To release our inner selves from the spiritual death that comes with living behind a facade designed to conform to external definitions of who and what we are.
> ~ Elisabeth Kubler-Ross

Near Death Experiences

The first written record of a *near-death experience (NDE)* – which occurs when an individual is dying from a serious illness or injury, or has died and is resuscitated - comes from the Greek philosopher Plato. In approximately 380 B.C., Plato wrote in *The Republic* about the NDE of a warrior named Er.

Some say that religious texts such as the Bible, the Tibetan Book of the Dead, and the Koran have describe NDEs which resemble modern reports. (Others dispute those interpretations.) Nonetheless, various surveys in the U.S. and other countries during the last few decades have found that anywhere from 4-15 percent of American adults report having had near-death experiences. There are many thousands NDE reports catalogued and studied, indicating that NDEs are much more common than were originally thought.

A pioneer of working with the dying and the stages of grief, Dr. Elizabeth Kubler-Ross collected twenty-thousand NDE reports with one of her colleagues. Based on her vast experience with them, Dr. Kubler-Ross claimed she had no doubt as to the genuineness of NDEs, or how deeply important these experiences were for the individuals.

In the early 1980s, a small article in the long-defunct *Brain-*

Mind Bulletin on NDE research caught my attention. From what I recall, this article described research that analyzed thousands of reports of NDEs from across the globe and that spanned several decades. These reports came from young children all the way to the very old. The analysis found that NDE reports could be reduced to eight characteristics, and although not everyone's NDE reflected all eight, they all had most of them.

At that time, the scientific community critiqued NDEs as some kind of fantasy fueled by movies and television. But the *Brain-Mind* article dispelled that idea because many of those NDE

What the dying have taught me:

Cultivate gratitude, surrender to reality, and shower the people you love with love.

The use of the word "cultivate" is important. A very wise man taught "We reap what we sow." And gratitude is magnetic. I have learned that those who can cultivate gratitude continue to find more things to be grateful for. Conversely, those who cultivate ingratitude seem to find more things to bitch about. The choice of attitude is ours – and that choice makes all the difference in the state of our own happiness.

By "surrender to reality" I mean accepting things as they are not as we wish them to be. The folks who refuse to accept their terminal situation generally have more pain and chaos as the end draws near. Accepting reality, living in the moment, savoring each precious second of life is rich living indeed.

~ Fred Grewe, Hospice Chaplain

reports were from people never exposed to Western media, with some of the experiences occurring before the advent of television. At this juncture – and more than thirty years after that small article passed my way – we still do not know what causes NDEs; the research is incomplete.

Many scientists claim that at impending death certain chemicals are released and that is what causes NDEs. If so, then we should have heard many, many more of these experiences since they would have been the rule and not the exception. Scientific explanations that focus on brain chemicals or label NDEs as "hallucinations" are often used to dismiss these reports, and later research has yet to prove these claims. Furthermore, NDE critiques are also not in keeping with a true scientific approach which requires an open, curious, and observant mind that is willing to consider new information, even if it upends our world view.

It's also clear that NDEs are important and even life-changing for the experiencer. As a clinician, that latter quality is enough to lead me and other clinicians to consider that NDEs have therapeutic value, even if only for a minority of individuals. In addition, if many people report similar life experiences, then there is some truth there, and their reports shouldn't be dismissed because they don't fit current ideas or certain types of research.

Through the last several decades, I've read many NDE reports and research, something which came in handy when some of my elderly residents asked me about their NDEs. With that in mind, let's see if NDEs can teach us a little something we can use to enhance our lives.

NDE Qualities

Based on the thousands of NDEs studied worldwide, it's now said that a NDE is unique to the experiencer and reflects their psychology, culture, and religious orientation. Not every NDE has every element listed below; and no single element is found in every NDE.

The most common NDE feature involves *intense feelings of peace, joy, love, and often, meeting an unconditionally loving light.*

The currently listed main features of reported NDEs are:

- A sense of being outside one's body; with the affected person even seeing medical efforts to revive the body.

- Sensation of rapid movement through darkness or a tunnel, often toward an intelligent, brilliant and powerful light.

- A sense of being in a different realm or landscapes. There may be encounters with deceased loved ones, animals, nonphysical heavenly beings and/or religious figures with whom communication is mind-to-mind. These figures may seem consoling, loving, or in some cases, terrifying.

- A sense of a border that once crossed offers no return back to human life. Sometimes there is a decision or a command to return to their body and live out the remainder of their life because it was not yet complete and there is more to learn.

- Receiving knowledge about the nature of life and the universe; or messages regarding their life's purpose or the future course of their life. Incredibly fast, clear thinking and understanding can also be present.

- Intense emotions, most often of profound peace, well-being, and unconditional love as well as a sense of oneness and interconnectedness with all life.

Sometimes, however, people report disturbing experiences marked by intense fear, confusion, guilt, horror, torment, or extreme loss. For example, one DNE experiencer wrote, "The 'hell' that I experienced was the pain, anguish, hurt and anger that I had caused others, or that I suffered as a result of my actions and words to others. 'Hell' was what I had created for myself and my own soul through turning my back on unconditional love, compassion and peace."

- A panoramic life review where the individual sees their life like a fast forwarding movie. They may relive past actions and how those actions hurt others. These life reviews do not include achievements and such. Rather, the focus is on the individual experiencing their emotional impact on others, and expanding their capacity to love.

As one can imagine, these experiences, whether joyous or frightening, will have an impact on the individual and how they view their life and proceed forward. Some residents have said they felt they had to return and complete some learning or mission, but they no longer feared death or going to hell. As a matter of fact, they looked forward to dying and the experience of unconditional love and peace, feeling our earthly existence was where suffering and ignorance dwelt.

After more than forty years of NDE research, respected psychiatrist Raymond Moody has been asked what he thinks happens at death. Dr. Moody answered:

> I think we enter into another stage of existence or another state of consciousness that is so extraordinarily different from the reality we have here in the physical world that the language we have is not yet adequate to describe this other state of existence or consciousness. Based on what I have heard from thousands of people, we enter into a realm of joy, light, peace, and love in which we discover that the process of knowledge does not stop when we die. Instead, the process of learning and development goes on for eternity.

> **Hell is...**
>
> During my near-death experience I had a descent into what you might call Hell, and it was very surprising. I did not see Satan or evil. My descent into Hell was a descent into each person's customized human misery, ignorance, and darkness of not knowing.
>
> It seemed like a miserable eternity. But each of the millions of souls around me had a little star of light always available. [N]o one seemed to pay attention to it. They were so consumed with their own grief, trauma and misery.
>
> [A]fter what seemed an eternity, I started calling out to that Light, like a child calling to a parent for help. Then the Light opened up and formed a tunnel that came right to me and insulated me from all that fear and pain… The Light came to me and turned into a huge golden angel….
>
> Then I was taken to the Light.
>
> ~ Mellen-Thomas Benedict

Moving Forward

Throughout time, every civilization has asked, "What is death? What happens when we die? Where do we go? How can I ensure a successful 'crossing' or a better life here so I won't end up in some kind of hell?"

Many cultures developed mythologies and doctrines to

answer these and other questions about death, but of course, no one knows for sure what happens. NDE reports could well be the closest thing we have to getting some information, so let us use one aspect of these experiences for our own benefit in the here and now.

Imagine a panoramic life review from the perspective of love, taking care not to criticize, shame, or condemn ourselves in the process. None of us is perfect or saintly. We are doing this review to expand our capacity to love, and to become more aware of ourselves and others.

In a quiet time, free from distractions, begin with 4 - 4 breathing. When it feels right, set an intention to yourself *to be aware of and learn from your past actions*. Then imagine a quick life review. This can be done for your entire life or in segments or regarding a particular relationship.

Reflect on:

- *How have I hurt another with my thoughtless actions?*

- *How much love have I given others, and how much love have I withheld?*

    Focus on the emotional impact your actions have on others. *Can you see how a moment of selfishness, unkindness, or ignorance on your part hurt someone?*

    From there, think about what you need to do to make amends or change your way of life so you feel at peace and in alignment with your true self. Ask yourself:

- *What do I need to become more aware of?*

- *How can I change for the future?*

- *Do I wish to make amends to the person(s) I have hurt?*

If you wish to make amends to someone who is dead or no longer in your life, move forward and put out new behaviors and attitudes toward others, even someone you don't know and may never see again. Remember, the purpose is to learn and expand our love, compassion, and kindness.

> Death is simply a shedding of the physical body like the butterfly shedding its cocoon. It is a transition to a higher state of consciousness where you continue to perceive, to understand, to laugh, and to be able to grow.
> ~ Elisabeth Kubler-Ross

Grief

When we lose someone we love, we may feel overwhelmed by emotions we can't name, much less understand. We all grieve differently, and each loss is also different, the grieving process sometimes changing as we grow older and become more accustomed to aging and death.

In grief, there is the sense of enormous loss or emptiness; that something vital is missing in our lives. The course of our lives feels altered as we experience the permanency of our loved one's death.

If it's a parent who dies, it signifies the end of an era in our lives. We are no longer someone's child, and we now come face-to-face with our own mortality. We too shall die, and it's not in the distant future anymore. Some may feel as if they have lost their greatest anchor in life, the one who loved them the most and whom they could confide in. Others do not feel this sentiment, or may actually feel relief their elderly parent has passed on and no longer needs to be cared for. In addition, they are relieved they no longer need to witness the ongoing worsening of their parent's mind and physical form, something most find depressing, sorrowful, and even frightening.

If it's a spouse that dies, we may feel adrift in life without a partner we depended on more than we realized. There may be the accompanying loss of a social network or circle of friends. Widows or widowers may feel acutely the loss of a spouse who took care of finances and other household business or responsibilities. Often after many decades of marriage, the surviving spouse has to build a new life and handle new responsibilities. They are embarking on a single and solitary life at a time when they feel least able to forge ahead, much less want to.

If a child, whether young or mature, dies, the heartache can be tremendous and last a lifetime. There is often a feeling that it "…isn't right, parents shouldn't outlive their children." It's often a devastating loss filled with endless regrets, what ifs, sorrow, and loss of faith in life. Yet, somehow, we must move on, especially if there are other children and family responsibilities. And, sometimes it comes as a surprise that life continues on, unaffected by our losses and feelings, no matter how immense and all-encompassing.

Often, people relive and think about their loved one's last days or hours, focusing solely on how the person looked as their body deteriorated. This is understandable since the mind likes to focus on the negative since it has more emotional intensity. Thus, the mind mulls over tragedies, disappointments, and injustices endlessly, never solving anything yet creating more and more story about the event and how we feel. People will focus on their story of loss, repeating what a tragedy it is, how senseless death is, how bad they feel, and so on. *This will not serve us; it will only accentuate our pain and cause more suffering.* In addition, we are focusing on only a small portion of our loved one's life.

The body will deteriorate and die, that is its nature. Don't let our minds discard the preciousness of who they were by mindlessly focusing on their last days and moments of disease and physical failure. **Remember their death and dying within the context of their**

whole life and our entire experience of that individual.

Consequently, I suggest to grieving family members that they focus on the love they've shared with their loved one. In the end, this is what's most important.

If you begin feeling overtaken by grief, close your eyes and imagine your loved one in your heart. Feel the love you have for them and the love you felt from them – the love you shared. Instantly, you should begin to feel better, more complete, full and even happy, with no overpowering thoughts of loss. That is because you have reconnected to love, and love cannot die.

> Love liberates.
> ~ Maya Angelou

If you believe in an afterlife or what NDE experiencers have reported about death, then you believe you will see your loved ones, sometime, somewhere, in another realm or another form. As a result, there was meaning and purpose to their life, even if they and we did not know and cannot know what it is. Death cannot take meaning, purpose, and love away from us.

And if you don't believe in any such accounts? No problem: Be a true scientist and keep an open mind; we'll all find out one day. Or, in the alternative, read some quantum physics for a mind-shaking perspective on the nature of life.

If your grieving does not end at some point, and you have fallen into depression or your life is spinning out of control, please consult a healthcare professional or psychotherapist. There is no reason to suffer needlessly, so explore other possibilities such as those listed in the Resources section or attend a grief support group at your local hospice or senior center. There might be something new and unexpected that can help you find peace with your loss.

> Don't grieve. Anything you lose comes round in another form.
> ~ Rumi

Time-Tested Tips

- What does your loved one want for end-of-life care? Are you willing and able to abide by their preferences even if they go against your own?

    There have been instances where a spouse or other relative tore up a resident's Advanced Directives or disregarded their preferences because they could not accept their decline and approaching death. Then they demanded more and more treatment, at times painful and uncomfortable, in order to keep the resident alive.

    If you were the resident, what would you want? What would you want your spouse or care manger to know before they had to make a medical decision on your behalf? If you were the responsible family member, what would you do in the face of your own fear and grief?

- What do you want for yourself? Have your wishes been documented and communicated to family or other responsible adult(s), including your doctor?

    If you don't know what you want or where to begin, visit Five Wishes at www.agingwithdignity.org.

- Are you satisfied with your life? Do you have any of the top five regrets of the dying? If so, what are you going to do so you don't die in a bog of regret and guilt?

- Did you create an imaginary life review? If so, what did you learn about yourself and your capacity to love?

- Like with any computer or smart device, are you updating your software, e.g., updating your old patterns of beliefs regarding life, death, others, yourself, and your way of living?

- Have you practiced your 4 - 4 Breathing, even as your loved one is approaching death? I sat with my parents as they were dying, practicing slow and gentle 4 - 4 breathing. Counting the inhales and exhales to four kept me in the moment and prevented my mind from spinning on itself. This was a sacred time, and I needed to respect that for them as well as for myself.

> There's no decision in death.
> People who know that there's no hope are free.
> The decision is out of their hands.
> It has always been that way, but some people have to die bodily to find out.
> No wonder they smile on their deathbeds.
> Dying is everything they were looking for in life.
> Their delusion of being in charge is over.
> When there's no choice, there's no fear.
> And in that, there is peace.
> They realize that they're home and that they've never left.
> ~ Byron Katie

Chapter 11
Healthy Aging

"It just sneaks up on you." Eyes twinkling, she smiled broadly, and with a wag of her finger added, "Don't grow old!"

"How do I do that?" I asked the lively centenarian, always the life of any party.

She shrugged one shoulder coquettishly and ambled down the hall to her painting class.

I've been told not to grow old countless times, as well as ordered to live life fully, but no one has ever told me how put off old age. The truth is no one knows, yet the hundred-year-olds don't seem to care. They never believed what they heard about old age, often saying, "It's just a number." These healthy minded old-olds have a zest for life, and don't complain about their ills or sit idle waiting for death. They're active in one way or another, engaged with life even as their bodies grow weak and they can no longer walk.

> If you're alive, there's a purpose for your life.
> ~ Rick Warren

Research into the old-old, including those over a hundred, has found several key traits we can cultivate at any age and take with us as we age. The number one characteristic for healthy aging is not health or wealth, but **flexibility**, the ability to change and adapt to life. Elders possessing this trait regularly bounce back from setbacks and losses. They did not allow negative events to diminish their satisfaction with life, or their inner sense of worth. In fact, they accepted obstacles as a natural part of life that we meet and move forward from.

If we look back at the last century, we can see these individuals experienced immeasurable, even horrific, world events and personal loses, yet they carried on – and somehow remained optimistic. They did not let negative emotions run their lives, and enjoyed laughter and the company of others. These centenarians also reported a spiritual perspective of some kind helped them navigate their way through life.

In addition, the centenarians continued to be as self-sufficient as possible and even creative, still learning despite cognitive aging and waning memory. They continued to derive pleasure and satisfaction from daily activities. They lived life as it presented itself to them and found enjoyment and meaning in everyday living. As a result, they felt everyday life is naturally meaningful.

Let's borrow a page from these hundred-year-olds and ask ourselves, "What qualities of theirs can we cultivate today?"

How can I be even more flexible and adaptable in life?

How can I cultivate even more laughter and fellowship today?

How can I encourage more creativity and learning today?

What small step can I take right now to nurture a positive attitude toward life?

The Golden Years or the Rusty Years?

The elusive American dream once included a retirement filled with "Golden Years." Research has shown that the most satisfying decade is our seventies, followed by the eighties.

However, that first wave of Twentieth Century retirees grew too old and their bodies aged past those golden years and into the rusty years. As of this writing, there are approximately 6.3 million old-olds in their rusty years who are eighty-five and above.

There are also approximately 65 million Baby Boomers (born: 1946-1964) still alive, with 38 million of those Boomers being female, and 28 million of these women being single. It's projected that three million Boomers will retire every year for the next twenty years, so by the year 2050 there will be an estimated *18 million old-old*.

Boomers are also referred to as the "sandwich generation" because some are helping elderly parents as well as adult children. Boomer women comprise the majority of caregivers for the elderly, and they often leave the workforce – something that impacts their earnings, and later, Social Security benefits. This will have long-term implications for them as well as society, especially since women live longer and have a greater risk for dementia.

Research also tells us that 80 percent of older adults have at least one chronic condition while 50 percent have two ailments. As a result, when we look forward to the coming years, we expect to see more and more old-old individuals, mostly women, who will need assistance of one kind or another.

Moreover, researchers who study risk factors for age-related diseases point out two broad categories. First, is **our genetic factors or predispositions** – something we can do nothing about. These are difficult to assess, and any research is still in its early stages. Scientists also tell us that although our genetic blueprint is fixed, its expression is switched on or off, or intensified, by outside influences. This opens the door to untold possibilities.

The second category is called **our modifiable risk factors**. These are the lifestyle factors we can change to substantially lessen their influence over our lives. In so doing, we'll find more keys to those sought after golden years as well as lessen the sting of those rusty years.

Let's review the recommendations of the Institute of Medicine (IOM) report on *Cognitive Aging* as well as other research about lifestyle factors.

> Mostly getting old is boring. I hate the stiffness in the bones. I was physically arrogant for years. I don't like it now that I have difficulty getting around. But a certain equanimity sets in, a certain detachment. Things seem less desperately important than they once did, and that's a pleasure.
> ~ Doris Lessing

What We Can Do

The most important steps to improve our health and aging are listed below. These actions are based on the latest research and the IOM's *Cognitive Aging* report, with my amplification. This is meant to spur you to improve your lifestyle and avoid the common pitfalls of aging; it is not a "prescription" for all people in all circumstances. Remember, the information in this book does not take the place of medical evaluation, treatment or recommendations. Do your own research in order to make choices that work for you.

These healthy steps include:

- **The human body was meant to move**. As a result, on a regular basis, be physically active and exercise so that it raises your heart rate to a moderate level for thirty minutes a day.

- **Reduce any cardiovascular risk factors such as high blood pressure, cholesterol, and diabetes.** Lose weight if you are obese or overweight. Stop smoking. Stop or at least significantly decrease alcohol and drug usage. However, low alcohol consumption such as a small glass of (red) wine is acceptable.

- **Be socially and intellectually active.** Be interested in others and in life. This will reduce isolation and loneliness, which are linked to depression. If you do feel depressed, please consult your doctor or a mental health professional; you needn't suffer in silence.

- **Continue to learn and exercise your brain with stimulating activities.** *Neuroplasticity*, the brain's ability to form new connections and compensate for injury and disease, continues throughout the life cycle. No matter our age, we have the potential to strengthen our cognitive abilities. Furthermore, increased education has been linked to less cognitive decline and reduced dementia. The recommendation is clear: *Exercise the mind, and make learning a lifelong habit.*

- **Consider learning a meditation practice such as mindfulness meditation.** Research has found doing so will not only help lower stress, but improve brain connectivity – and that means less cognitive decline. (For stress reduction, consider the mindfulness-based program at www.MindfulLivingPrograms.com. Check the Resources in the Appendix for other possibilities.) Also, *don't forget to consciously breathe.* Make 4 - 4 Breathing a part of your life.

- **Manage medications well.** Regularly review them with your physician to avoid side effects or impaired mental abilities. If you have any medical conditions, manage them as well as possible with regular consultation with your healthcare providers.

- **Get adequate sleep.** If you have any sleep problems, consult a professional.

- **Make dietary changes so you are eating a healthier diet.** Limit or cut out sugars and simple carbohydrates; fried and fast foods; soft drinks and other sugary drinks; products with high fructose corn syrup; bread and other baked goods; processed fats; and dairy foods.

If we look back at those old-olds and centenarians mentioned above, we will find they ate a much simpler and healthier diet than the modern American diet. Today's major "killers" are "lifestyle-related" diseases we can take steps to avoid, minimize, or at least better manage. Dr. Michael Roizen of Cleveland Clinic's Wellness Institute, adds, "Dietary choices alone can make you 13 years younger or older than your actual age."

The most recommended diet for healthy hearts and minds and to lower inflammation is some version of the Mediterranean Diet. In other words, eat more lean protein like fish (contains Omega-3 fatty acids) and chicken, and use olive oil. Eat lots of vegetables, leafy greens, and fruits, including blueberries which have been found to aid mental abilities. Also, eat avocados, nuts, seeds, legumes, and grains (non-gluten preferably). Lastly, learn to read food labels so you know what you're eating. (For more information, visit MayoClinic.org and ClevelandClinic.org, among other websites.)

- **Avoid or at least minimize "risky behaviors."** These are behaviors and activities we may have once engaged in safely, but with increasing age they pose a threat to our well-being and independence.

Here are a few examples to highlight this issue. A seventy-five-year-old climbs on his roof to do a repair, something he's done for decades, but slips and falls, never to walk again. Or an eighty-year-old with a "bad back" who continues to play golf after back surgery, dismissing his doctor's warning and his own pain. Or consider the seventy-eight-year-old Florida "snowbird" who drove back and forth to her winter home despite cognitive and physical decline that made a long drive alone increasingly dangerous for herself as well as others.

A risky behavior can also be an activity that's less obviously demanding such as gardening, bicycling, walking the dog, and so on. With advancing age, unsteady balance, and possibly the effect of old injuries, surgeries or medications, previous pastimes can now become risky and need to be re-evaluated. Invariably when these seniors are asked about continuing these pursuits, they say, "But I've always done it," forgetting their bodies have changed, perhaps significantly. So be smart about what you choose to do so you don't pay a hefty, an unnecessary price.

- **Tackle stress and psychological patterns that affect immune functioning and well-being, including changing all attitudes and beliefs that do not support well-being and happiness.** Do so even if you are physically active, eat right, and follow all the previous recommendations. As cell biologist Dr. Bruce Lipton has said, our beliefs, including our beliefs about aging, will affect our stem cell functioning and lead to either regeneration or decline due to negative thinking and negative self-talk.

It's also important to keep in mind that it's easier to change our attitudes and habits when we're younger than it is to wait until old age and illness. If we wait until we have to change our ways, then our attitudes and beliefs can be so ingrained, and our capabilities so compromised, this it is difficult, if not impossible, to change.

To live better, cultivate self-compassion, happiness, and the qualities of the hundred-year-olds. Spend time with nature, even if that only means sitting on your back porch. Cultivate interest in life, creativity. Build a spiritual foundation that both supports you and answers the bigger questions in life. This is not to say you'll find answers to all of life's questions, chances are you won't. So learn to accept and enjoy the mysteries of life.

> The web of life both cradles us and calls us to weave it further.
> ~ Joanna Macy

How we live our remaining years is our choice, and we can make choices that will enhance our well-being right now and into the future. We needn't wait for some future time or for others to join or approve our efforts and choices. The last chapter of our lives need not be painfully short or long, or devoid of love and meaning. As with nature and its seasons, the winter of our lives can be a beautiful and nurturing time, full of opportunity. We can start by supporting and cherishing our daily life with the practice of gratitude.

> Gratitude unlocks the fullness of life. It turns what we have into enough, and more. It turns denial into acceptance, chaos to order, confusion to clarity. It can turn a meal into a feast, a house into a home, a stranger into a friend. Gratitude makes sense of our past, brings peace for today, and creates a vision for tomorrow.
> ~ Melody Beattie

Gratitude

Gratitude is an attitude toward life whereby we recognize the good, however small and inconsequential, yet do not deny or minimize the negative. When we value what we have, we begin recognizing each moment as unique. When each moment is unique, our existence seems brighter, more complete, and our perspective less problematic.

Intentionally cultivating gratitude results in:

- increased health and well-being;
- greater happiness, energy and optimism;
- sounder sleep;
- more compassion, generosity; and
- more satisfying, kinder and loving relationships.

Gratitude is linked to less fear, anxiety, and depression, as well as a decreased tendency to get angry and hostile when provoked or triggered. When we have an attitude of gratitude toward life, there is little room for resentment, criticism, jealously, and negative comparisons of ourselves to others. In sum, grateful individuals show increased life satisfaction, and with that comes greater peace, health, forgiveness, and a sense of fulfillment.

Psychologist Robert Emmons, who has studied gratitude at length, says,

> We all begin life dependent on others, and most of us end life dependent on others. If we are lucky, in between we have roughly 60 years or so of unacknowledged dependency. The human condition is such that throughout life, not just at the beginning and end, we are profoundly dependent on other people. …
>
> Gratitude is the truest approach to life. We did not create or fashion ourselves. We did not birth ourselves. Life is about giving, receiving, and repaying. We are receptive beings, dependent on the help of others, on their gifts and their kindness.

Cultivating gratitude takes a few moments each day. Not sure how to start? Begin by noticing something positive in your life, something or someone you are thankful for is in your life. For example, when you wake up, you can be grateful for the bed you slept in, the cat curled at your feet, the bird singing outside your window, the smell of coffee brewing, and so forth. For the rest of the day, make a point of noticing other small things, or events or people about which you are grateful. For example, be positively aware of the food you ate, the garbage men who hauled away the trash, the person who cleaned the public restroom you used, the breath you were able to take unimpeded, and so on.

Consider keeping a gratitude journal to keep you focused on what's good and positive in your life. In short order, you'll begin to reap the benefits of gratitude.

> If you want to see the brave, look at those who can return love for hatred. If you want to see the heroic, look for those who can forgive.
> ~ Bhagavad Gita

The End is Always a Beginning

It may have been difficult for you, as well as others, to read and contemplate this book at many moments. Some of the examples and issues are heartrending. So how can we be grateful about these happenings? One way to view them is that they also point us toward a better, fuller, and more realistic way of being in life.

Consider the stories that can be viewed as gloomy or even alarming. While our first reaction is to push them all away, for most of us much of the information they present will have been new – *and in that lies opportunity for further change and growth, more joy, and greater empowerment as we grow older.*

> Forgiveness is not an occasional act: it is an attitude.
> ~ Martin Luther King, Jr.

Whenever we take time to review our life and our choices, challenges will emerge that are seldom for the faint-hearted or those who want swift and easy answers. Life doesn't work that way; at least it never has in my life. Life will nudge us, coax us along, and in the end demand we be more than we think we're capable of. Life will push us to go beyond our limited stories about whom and what we are, to travel beyond the legacy of our parents, culture, and our enduring habits and beliefs. At that fork in the road, we'll need to go within for a deeper communion with our true self, and then step outward with the gentle expression of our true nature.

In the face of most of what you've read, do not assume getting old is a one-way trek into greater and greater decline and loss with no redeeming features. That's not what the healthy minded old-old tell us. Yes, the body declines and we'll have to give up favorite activities or do them differently, but our spirit and love can shine undiminished until our last breath on this earth. And if you do suffer from aches and pains or more significant illnesses, remember you are more than your physical body and all of your doing, and much more than your mind with its repetitive thoughts and stories.

In the silence of the space in between your thoughts, and within the spaciousness of your breath, rediscover over and over again your beingness within the dance of life.

> Each today, well-lived, makes yesterday a dream of
> happiness and each tomorrow a vision of hope. Look,
> therefore, to this one day, for it and it alone is life.
> ~ Sanskrit poem

Appendix

Checklists

Below are two Checklists: **Rehab/Skilled Nursing** and **Long-Term Care.** These checklists highlight the most important care issues in rehab, nursing homes, and ALFs. There is some repetition because some items overlap to ensure each checklist is as complete as possible. Since every individual and every situation is unique and will change over time, feel free to add or modify the checklist(s). Keep in mind that solutions are not often immediately apparent, especially the result we think should happen or when it should happen. As a result, it's beneficial to cultivate patience, compassion, and acceptance of change and life as it is.

Do not hesitate to do your own research to find what works best for you and your loved one, and do not be afraid to ask questions. That said, do not expect clear and definitive answers from facility doctors and staff early on since they may not know the resident well enough, and for many questions there are no clear cut answers. In addition, realize that answers change as the patient's health changes and/or their dementia increases. Also, healthcare professionals and facilities must abide by confidentially laws so they should never disclose confidential patient information unless you are legally authorized to receive this information.

Rehab refers to residents in a skilled nursing facility for rehabilitation following a hospitalization or an inpatient rehab admission. Since rehab residents are transferred from a hospital or may be hospitalized during their rehab or long-term care stay, the Rehab Checklist includes issues seen in a hospital setting. Finally, please do not use the Checklists without first reading this book because you will miss important information that will help you better understand and manage these situations.

Rehab/Skilled Nursing Checklist

- What are the discharge and transfer arrangements to the rehab/skilled nursing facility from the hospital or other setting? What time? (Hospital discharges are usually late morning into the afternoon, but can be late into the evening.)

- Did the transfer to the nursing home/rehab center go well? If possible, it's best if a family member or trusted friend is waiting for the resident. There is a great deal for the resident to get used to in the first few hours and days. In addition, a ride in an ambulance or transport van is often bumpy and stressful, even painful.

- Remind the resident where they are and what the purpose is. Chances are they'll need to be reminded again and again. If they do not like the word "nursing home," use rehab center or something similar they can accept.

- The new resident will be evaluated by Rehab as well as other departments, beginning with Nursing as soon as possible following their transfer and admission. All these **required** evaluations can overwhelm the resident who feels as if they are being bombarded by questions and people. They still do not feel well and probably cannot keep track of what's happening or what others are telling them.

- Has the resident's skin been checked lately? If the resident developed a skin tear, pressure ulcer, bed sore or wound in the hospital, it's extremely important they are turned regularly. Some residents do not like this because it can be uncomfortable to lay on one side or the other, but it is necessary to avoid the wound becoming very large and deep, and very painful. Any questions, please discuss with nursing.

Bed sores in the elderly can develop **quickly**, and are painful and slow to heal. Bed sores occur most often in the general tailbone area and heels. Sometimes the resident will need to see a wound specialist and have a "wound vac" placed on the wound. Heel sores often need booties or heels lifted off the bed.

- Get to know the facility and your resident's primary staff as well as others involved in their stay such as Admissions, Social Services, Business Office, etc.

- Rehab will begin as soon as possible, starting with one or more evaluations. Some residents do not feel up to this, but they are necessary and required by Medicare and other insurance.

- Once they begin rehab therapy, gently encourage the resident since rehab is essential to their recovery. Don't nag, criticize or scold; that will be stressful and counterproductive. Don't attend rehab unless their therapist requested your presence.

- Diagnosis? What is the primary problem? Additional or secondary problems?

- What is the preliminary treatment plan? If specialists are involved, when is the next appointment(s)?

REHAB/SKILLED NURSING CHECKLIST

- What are the projected rehab goals and length of stay? Keep in mind that there will not be a tentative discharge date until the resident is much closer to their goals.

- What is the prognosis? (Projection as to course of illness and treatment; best and worst case scenarios if applicable.)

- What medical decisions need to be made now? In the near future?

  Does the patient have a Living Will, (Durable) Power of Attorney, DNR (Do Not Resuscitate if heart stops), Healthcare Surrogate? These are Florida terms and forms; other states will differ. Consult an attorney regarding legal issues.

- What do you need to tell and discuss with the patient? Are they alert enough to understand? Make it simple and concrete to aid understanding. Most family members say too much, often in an unfocused way. This leads to confusion and even arguments. It's helpful to first write out what you want to communicate to help you focus on the main issues.

  Involve other family members? Information and updates only, or for inclusion in decision-making? Who? Contact information?

  If the resident cannot express their wishes, what would they want if they could tell you? Who would they like to be called and for what purpose, e.g., updates or decision-making involvement?

- Medications – Make a list and track changes.

    Side effects? Allergies? (Petite, elderly women are often prone to side effects.)

    What has been discontinued? Any psychotropic or anti-depressant medications discontinued in the hospital? If the resident has a mental health history, please make sure the facility knows that information, including medications in the recent past.

    Alcohol and/or Street Drugs? If the patient has an alcohol and/or drug history, please tell the doctor or nurse. If their use is recent or long term, it's possible they are detoxing, and this will affect their mental abilities and their participation in rehab.

    Any sedating drugs such as anti-anxiety medications (Xanax, Ativan, Restoril, among others)? Xanax or generic Alprazolam for anxiety is a muscle relaxant that has been shown to contribute to falls in the elderly and its use in nursing homes should be monitored.

    Antibiotics? These can make the elderly patient feel "spacey" or out of it, upset their stomach or decrease appetite and taste, etc.

    Anesthesia for recent surgery? For the elderly, anesthesia can make them look as if they have significant dementia when they do not. Tell the patient if they're worried about their cognitive or memory lapses that this will pass over time (usually 3-8 weeks). However, be aware that for a very small percentage, a cognitive decline can be permanent.

- Eating enough? Do they need special food items? Protein shakes, bars, or ice cream? Check with Nursing and/or Dietary. If you bring in food, bring in something the patient likes, smells good, in small amounts, but always in keeping with any dietary restrictions.

- Drinking enough water? Fluid restriction? Need liquids thickened? Many residents do not like the taste or texture of thickened liquids, however, this prevents choking. If the resident insists on drinking regular water, discuss this with nurse or dietician.

- Pain? Where? When? Are pain medications controlling their pain enough?

- Agitated? Restless? Aggressive? Uncooperative? Slow or sudden onset? Is the cause known? What, if any, medications are being used to control these behaviors?

- If your loved one has **dementia** or is newly diagnosed, educate yourself as to what to expect and how best respond to them. Don't expect them to be the person they once were or how you think they should be. Remind yourself that dementia is a progressive brain disease, so they are not in control of their thinking, memory, reactions, and impulses as they once might have been. (See the Resources section.)

- Has there been a significant decline in mental abilities or personality changes? Confusion, disorientation, don't know where they are or what's happening, impaired memory, delusions (believing things that aren't true), hallucinations (seeing things others can't see), paranoia, depression, crying, anxiety, fear, and so on.

- Delirium? A sudden impairment in mental abilities and can include inability to focus, poor memory and speech, confusion, agitation, combativeness, hallucinations, delusions, and extreme emotions. Or, their metal status can fluctuate with periods of withdrawal with little or no activity and responsiveness. Talk to their nurse, Nurse Practitioner, or attending physician. If possible, provide a history regarding the resident's functioning before admission.

- Sudden confusion and mental decline? Ask about a UTI (Urinary Tract Infection), but remember there are other reasons for a mental decline including the ups and downs of dementia as well as its progression. As always, consult with a physician.

- Poor Safety awareness such as trying to get up and falling, pulling out IVs and other lines to equipment, swatting away help, and so similar behaviors.

- Is the resident sleeping fairly well? Some residents need special mattresses or are not sleeping due to pain, side effects, anxiety, noisy roommate(s), lights, or room temperature.

- Is the patient complaining about anything? What is the complaint? Investigate to determine how accurate or significant it is, or whether it's due to unrealistic expectations. If needed, be their advocate and go to the appropriate staff member such as a nurse manager, social worker, etc. (Consult Chapter 7 regarding complaints.)

- Glasses and/or hearing aids? Where are they? These are easily misplaced in a facility, ambulance or other

REHAB/SKILLED NURSING CHECKLIST

transport. If the patient is not wearing their glasses, they may feel confused and vulnerable if they cannot see what is going on around them. Without their hearing aids they may not hear what others are saying and will be prone to suspiciousness, distrust, and lack of cooperation.

- What can you bring to make them more comfortable? Ask the patient, and keep it simple. Do they need clothing, shoes, or other items from home? Don't bring expensive or special items that can be lost or damaged in the facility laundry.

- If the resident if not adjusting well and is exhibiting psychological symptoms such as depression, anxiety, worry, crying, angry outbursts, etc. and/or they are not participating in rehab, request a consult with a psychologist.

- Visitors: Make sure the patient is up for company and visitors do not stay long if that tires the patient. Don't rely on the patient to tell visitors they're tired and visitors ought to leave. Also, limit the amount of sugary snacks as well as plants and flowers. (Do not expect staff to care for the flowers and plants, or residents to curb a sweet tooth.)

- Do not expect the rehab resident to attend Activities. Their number one priority is to do rehab and recover, not socialize. Toward the end of their rehab when they are feeling much better, some residents choose to attend Activities after they've completed their rehab therapies. At that point, Activities is a positive.

- Insurance and financial issues. Are these being taken care of?

- Discharge Planning: the social worker or other assigned staff will contact resident and/or responsible family member when it's time to plan for discharge.

  In Florida, a regularly scheduled Care Plan Conference will be held to review the resident's progress and status, discharge date, etc. The resident and/or responsible family member(s) will be invited to attend.

  Sometimes due to special medical needs, the resident maybe transferred to an "inpatient rehab" or a "complex care" facility. Facility staff will discuss this with the resident and/or family member/legal representative.

  Going home? What do they need? Home Health? The facility's discharge planner will take care of these issues, and discuss them with resident and/or responsible family member.

  Do they need to go into an ALF or a Long-Term Care nursing home? Visit potential facilities if possible.

  At the appropriate time, tell the patient what the discharge plan is, and briefly, the reasons for the plan. Do not expect them to remember, so keep it simple and repeat as necessary. Remind them that you (or other family member, caregiver, or friend) will be with them and they are not alone.

- Take care of yourself: eat healthy, drink plenty of water, rest, and practice 4 - 4 Breathing to calm yourself as well as create a peaceful atmosphere in your loved one's room. If you are an elderly spouse, the ongoing stress of your resident's health crisis and rehab will slowly impact your health, so take good care of yourself. Also be sure to maintain regular check-ups with your physician.

Remind yourself that the beginning of rehab is always difficult and uncertain. You need to take it one moment at a time, one day at a time, and see how the recovery proceeds. Not every decision needs to be made today. You are also not responsible to solve every problem perfectly or take away your loved one's pain and suffering.

You will have to learn to accept limitations and imperfection. This includes the resident's limitations such as their advanced age, condition of their body, reactions to medications, treatments, and rehab; personality, mental abilities, and attitude (some people are better at being a patient than others), as well as the limitations of family members (some will be helpful while others not at all). You will also face the limitations of medicine and the medical staff; the facility; government and insurance regulations; and last but not least, your own limitations. Be kind to yourself, especially during this challenging time.

Long-Term Care Checklist

- If possible, prepare your loved one for transfer to long-term care in a nursing home. Consider using some of the options presented in the long-term care chapters.

- Manage your guilt and doubt using the suggestions in **Getting Older, Being Here**.

- Did the transfer to the long-term nursing home go well? If possible, it's best if a family member or trusted friend is waiting for the resident. There is a great deal for the resident to get used to in the first few hours and days. In addition, a ride in an ambulance or transport van is often bumpy and stressful, even painful.

- Remind the resident where they are and what the purpose is using language they can understand and hopefully accept. Chances are they'll need to be reminded again, but sometimes once is enough if the resident does not like to be reminded.

- The new resident will be evaluated by various departments in a new nursing home, beginning with Nursing as soon as possible following their admission. Sometimes all these **required** evaluations are overwhelming and annoying to the new resident because they've been through it before, and they don't want to be there anyway.

  If the resident is staying in the same facility and transitioning into long-term care, the transfer will be more seamless. However, they may have to adjust to a new roommate, unit, and care team.

- Has the resident's skin been checked lately? Skin tears, pressure ulcers, bed sores and wounds in the elderly infirmed patient can develop **quickly**, and are painful and slow to heal. Bed sores occur most often in the general tailbone area and heels, and require the resident to be turned regularly or pressure on the heels relieved.

- Get to know the new nursing home or unit and your resident's primary nursing staff. This often includes Admissions, Social Services, Business Office, etc. If there's a problem, it's best to go directly to the responsible staff. Often, family members or residents will address requests and complaints to an aide (CNA) or housekeeper who is not responsible for that issue and may forget to pass it along to the right person.

  If your loved one or you have an issue with a roommate or another resident, please refrain from approaching the resident or their family. It's best to address these problems and complaints with the appropriate staff or manager.

- Once a rehab resident transitions into long-term care, rehab is terminated. However, the resident may receive "Restorative Therapy" or something similar. Gently encourage them to participate since restorative therapy is important to maintain their mobility, strength, lessen pain, etc. Check with the facility about this service since it will vary among facilities, as well as whether the resident qualifies.

  Do not attend restorative therapy with your loved one unless their therapist or restorative aide has requested your attendance.

- Diagnosis? What is the primary problem? Additional or secondary problems?

- If your loved one has **dementia** or is newly diagnosed, educate yourself as to what to expect and how to best respond to them. Don't expect them to be the person they once were or how you think they should be since their brain has already undergone significant changes and will continue to deteriorate. (See the Resources section.)

- What is the preliminary treatment plan? If specialists are involved, when is the next appointment(s)?

- What medical decisions need to be made now? In the near future?

Does the patient have a Living Will, (Durable) Power of Attorney, DNR (Do Not Resuscitate if heart stops), Healthcare Surrogate? These are Florida terms and forms; other states will differ. Consult an attorney regarding legal issues.

Lastly, it is helpful to make funeral or cremation arrangements as soon as possible. Then when the time comes, all that is needed is a phone call by the facility and family can attend to other matters as well as their own grief.

- What do you need to tell and discuss with the patient? Are they alert enough to understand? Make it simple and concrete. If you want to know whether they understand, ask them to repeat what they've heard and what options are available for a particular issue or decision that needs to be made.

If the resident cannot express their wishes, what would the patient want if they could tell you? What have they said in the past? Who would they like to be called and for what purpose, e.g., updates or decision-making involvement?

Involve other family members? Information and updates only, or for inclusion in any decision-making? Who? Contact information?

- Medications – Make a list and track changes.

  Side effects? Allergies? (Petite, elderly women are often prone to side effects.)

  What has been discontinued? Any psychotropic or anti-depressant medications discontinued during a recent hospital stay? If the resident has a mental health history, make sure the facility knows that information, including medications in the recent past.

  Alcohol and/or Street Drugs? If the patient has an alcohol and/or drug history, tell the doctor or nurse. If their use is recent or long-term, they maybe detoxing and this will affect their mental abilities and possibly their participation in Rehab, treatments, etc.

  Any sedating drugs such as anti-anxiety medications? (Xanax, Ativan, Restoril, among others) Xanax or generic Alprazolam for anxiety is a muscle relaxant that has been shown to contribute to falls in the elderly, so its use in nursing homes should be monitored.

  Anti-psychotics? These are prescribed for extreme agitation, combativeness, paranoia, hallucinations, etc.

These can affect the elderly to a greater degree and must be monitored.

Antibiotics? These may make the elderly patient feel "spacey" or out of it, upset their stomach or decrease appetite and taste, etc.

Anesthesia for recent surgery? For the elderly, anesthesia can make them look as if they have significant dementia when they do not. Tell the patient if they're worried that this effect will pass over time (usually 3-8 weeks). However, be aware that for a very small percentage, this mental decline can be permanent.

- Eating enough? Do they need any special food items? Eating too much sugar? Do they need protein shakes, bars, or ice cream? Check with Nursing and/or Dietary.

  If you bring in food, bring in something the patient likes, smells good, in small amounts, but always in keeping with dietary restrictions.

- Drinking enough water? Fluid restriction? Need liquids thickened? Many residents do not like the taste or texture of thickened liquids, however, this helps prevent choking. If the resident insists on drinking water and other liquids without thickener, discuss this with the nurse or dietician.

- Alcohol? Some residents may be allowed to have alcoholic beverages they provide, but **only** with the doctor's consent. Street or recreational drugs are never allowed. Most nursing homes no longer allow **smoking** on their campuses. If smoking is allowed, it will only be in designated areas. If your loved one smokes, consider transferring them to a facility that allows smoking to avoid ongoing problems and power struggles.

- Pain? Where? When? Are pain medications controlling their pain enough?

- Are other services such as Podiatry, Dental, or Vision needed? Check with Social Services to see if these services are provided on-site.

- Agitated? Restless? Aggressive? Uncooperative? Slow or sudden onset? Is the cause known? What, if any, medications are being used to control these behaviors?

- Sudden confusion and mental decline? Ask about a UTI (Urinary Tract Infection), but remember there are other reasons for a mental decline including the ups and downs of dementia as well as its progression. As always, consult with a physician.

- Poor Safety Awareness? This includes trying to get up and falling, trying to dress, go to the bathroom, or get up from their wheel-chair when they are unable to do so, show unsteady balance and gait but refusing to use a walker, pulling out IVs and tubes, swatting away help, and so forth.

- Is the resident sleeping fairly well? Some patients need special mattresses or are not sleeping due to pain, anxiety, noisy roommate(s), light, or room temperature.

- Is the patient complaining about anything? What is the complaint?

    Who was involved? What happened or what was said? When and Where? Investigate to determine how accurate or significant it is, or whether it's due to an unrealistic expectation. If needed, be their advocate. (See Chapter 7.)

If the resident hates the facility and there is no practical way to resolve the problem(s) to their satisfaction, consider transfer to another facility. If the same complaints happen in every facility, then the resident is not adjusting or incapable of adjusting due to medical and/or cognitive diseases or unrealistic expectations. In this case, you have to realize you cannot make them happy and satisfied, and they may have to learn to "live with it." Consider a consult with a psychologist or psychiatrist.

- Glasses and/or hearing aids? Where are they? These are easily misplaced in a nursing home, and residents have been known to throw hearing aids away or place them on their meal tray, etc. If the patient is not wearing their glasses, they may feel confused if they cannot see what is going on around them. Without hearing aids, they may not hear what others are telling them and this results in suspiciousness, distrust, and lack of cooperation.

- What can you bring that might help them feel more comfortable? Ask the patient, and keep it simple. Do they need clothing, shoes, or other items from home?

- Don't nag, criticize, threaten, or scold. It's stressful and counterproductive.

- If the resident if not adjusting to their illness, placement, roommate, and/or exhibiting symptoms such as depression, anxiety, worry, crying, paranoia, refusing rehab and other treatments, etc., request a consult with a psychologist or psychiatrist.

Or, if you as a family member/care manager are experiencing stress regarding how to deal with your loved one or explain that they are not going home, etc., and would like to speak to someone, ask the social worker if the facility has a psychologist.

- Has there been a significant decline in mental abilities or personality changes? This includes confusion, disorientation, don't know where they are or what's happening, impaired memory, delusions (believing things that aren't true), hallucinations (seeing things others can't see), paranoia, depression, crying, anxiety, etc.

- Delirium? A sudden impairment in mental abilities and can include inability to focus, poor memory and speech, confusion, agitation, combativeness, delusions, hallucinations, and extreme emotions. Or, mental status can fluctuate with periods of withdrawal with little or no activity and responsiveness. Contributing factors include severe or chronic medical illness, infection, surgery, medication, drug and/or alcohol abuse. Speak to their nurse, Nurse Practitioner, or attending physician.

- Visitors: Make sure the patient is up for company and visitors do not stay long if visits tire or stress the patient. Don't rely on the patient to tell visitors they're tired and visitors ought to leave.

  Also, limit the amount of sugary snacks, gifts and flowers; and don't expect staff to care for the flowers and plants since space is limited. If possible, try to make their room or part of a room personal, assuming they like that.

- Not every long-term resident will want to attend Activities. Some prefer to be alone and quiet in their room, perhaps reading, watching TV or enjoying a hobby. Others are more social and would enjoy Activities. Suggest they attend a few Activities to see which ones they might like. If they prefer not to attend, let them be.

- Insurance and financial issues; what needs to be taken care of at this point?

- In Florida, regularly scheduled Care Plan Conferences will be held to review the resident's progress and status. The resident and/or responsible family member/care manager will be invited to attend. For some residents, especially those with dementia, etc., it's best if they do not attend if they become confused or stressed.

Residents have legal rights they can exercise while living in a nursing home, including the right to refuse medications, treatments, and/or activities. They also have the right to engage in consensual sexual relations in private. If you have any questions, please discuss them with the social worker.

- Discharge Planning: the social worker or other assigned staff will contact resident and/or responsible family member when it's time to plan for discharge.

Going home? What does the resident need? Discharge planning will discuss arrangements with the resident and/or family member.

At the appropriate time, tell the patient what the discharge plan is and briefly, the reasons for the plan. Don't expect them to remember, so keep it simple and repeat as necessary. Remind them that you (or other family member, friend) will be with them, if possible, and that they are not alone.

- Take care of yourself: eat healthy, drink plenty of water, rest, exercise, cultivate self-compassion, practice relaxation or centering techniques, and do something fun. Practice 4 - 4 Breathing to calm yourself as well as create a peaceful atmosphere in your loved one's room. If you are an elderly spouse, the ongoing stress of your loved one's health decline and long-term care placement will impact your health, so take extra good care of yourself. Also be sure to maintain regular check-ups with your physician.

The beginning of long-term placement is always difficult and your loved one's adjustment can take several months. You need to take it one moment at a time, one day at a time, and see how the situation develops. Not every decision needs to be made today. You are also not responsible to solve every problem perfectly or take away your loved one's pain and suffering, although the nursing home must call you if a problem or incident occurs. Be realistic in your expectations of your resident, their illness and decline, the facility, and yourself.

You will have to learn to accept limitations and imperfection. This includes the resident's limitations such as their advanced age, condition of their body, reactions to medications and treatments; personality, mental abilities, and attitude (some people are better at being a patient than others), as well as the limitations of family members (some will be helpful while others not). You will also face the limitations of medicine and the medical staff; the facility; government and insurance regulations; and last but not least, your own limitations. Be kind to yourself, especially during this challenging time that could last years.

Resources

The following recent books and websites are suggestions to help you explore topics related to **Getting Older, Being Here**. This is not an exhaustive list by any means; it's just a beginning. These resources represent different points of view so we may go beyond our "tried and true" and transform how we see life, aging, pain, illness, nursing homes, and the transition we call death. In addition, visit www.GettingOlderBeingHere.com for informative blogs.

Aging Well

- David Bernstein, MD ~ *I've Got Some Good News and Some Bad News: YOU'RE OLD: Tales of a Geriatrician, What to expect in your 60's, 70's, 80's, & Beyond*
- Joan Chittister ~ *The Gift of Years: Growing Older Gracefully*
- Kristy Clark ~ *Aging with Health: The Secrets to Healthy Aging and Making the Best of Your Golden Years*
- Rabbi Rachel Cowan and Dr. Linda Thal ~ *Wise Aging* (Recommended)
- David Perlmutter, MD ~ *The Grain Brain* www.drperlmutter.com
- Lewis Richman ~ *Aging as a Spiritual Practice: A Contemplative Guide to Growing Older and Wiser*
- Daniel Stevens ~ *Aging Well and Gracefully: How to Slow*

Down Aging and Enter Your Golden Years Well with Grace, Inner Peace & Become Wiser Naturally

- Andrew Weil, MD ~ *Healthy Aging: A Lifelong Guide to Your Well-Being*

Older Adults & Parents; Dementia and Alzheimer's

Information regarding dementia and Alzheimer's, whether online or other media, will differ depending on the year and country published, training, profession or role of the writer or presenter. These differences, including differences in symptoms, diagnostic labels, staging or levels, are typically minor if we keep in mind that what we know and how we handle the various dementias is still evolving. Moreover, each individual with dementia or Alzheimer's is unique.

It's important to remember that research regarding the "elderly" denotes men and women age sixty-five and up, and "old-old" means age eighty-five and up. As of this writing, research does *not* distinguish between younger seniors and those in their eighties, nineties, and beyond who have different bodies, needs, psychology and early conditioning, and respond differently to illness, traumas, treatments, surgery, and medications.

For more information regarding dementia and Alzheimer's disease, refer to Chapter 9. For information on how to age well and reduce the likelihood of dementia, see Chapter 11.

- Robert F. Bornstein, PhD and Mary A. Languirand, PhD ~ *When Someone You Love Needs Nursing Home, Assisted Living, or in-Home Care*
- Eleanor Feldman Barbera, PhD ~ *The Savvy Resident's Guide: Everything You Wanted to Know About Your Nursing*

RESOURCES

Home Stay but Were Afraid to Ask

- Jolene Brackey ~ *Creating Moments of Joy for the Person with Alzheimer's or Dementia: A Journal for Caregivers*
- Jennifer Ghent-Fuller ~ *Thoughtful Dementia Care: Understanding the Dementia Experience* www.understanding-dementia-experience.com (Recommended)
- Nancy L. Mace, MA and Peter V. Rabins, MD ~ *The 36-Hour Day: A Family Guide to Caring for People Who Have Alzheimer Disease, Related Dementias, and Memory Loss*
- Virginia Morris ~ *How to Care for Aging Parents, 3rd Edition: A One-Stop Resource for All Your Medical, Financial, Housing, and Emotional Issues*
- Amy Newmark and Angela T. Geiger ~ *Chicken Soup for the Soul: Living with Alzheimer's & Other Dementias*
- Daniel Potts, MD and Ellen Potts ~ *A Pocket Guide for the Alzheimer's Caregiver*
- Linda Rhodes ~ *The Essential Guide to Caring for Aging Parents*
- Susan Kiser Scarff and Ann Kiser Zultner ~ *Dementia: The Journey Ahead*
- www.TeepaSnow.com
- Paula Scott ~ *Surviving Alzheimer's: Practical tips & soul-saving wisdom for caregivers* (Recommended)
- David Solie ~ *How to Say It to Seniors*
- M.L. Wagner, MD ~ *Nursing Homes: Working, Living, and Dying*

End of Life & Grief; Near-Death Experiences (NDE)

- Martha Jo Atkins, PhD ~ *Shift Your Grief* (website) www.MarthaAtkins.com
- Maggie Callanan ~ *Final Gifts: Understanding the Special Awareness, Needs, and Communications of the Dying*
- *Five Wishes* www.agingwithdignity.org
- Atul Gawande, MD ~ *Being Mortal*
- Fred Grewe ~ *What the Dying Have Taught Me about Living: The Awful Amazing Grace of God*
- Martha W. Hickman ~ *Healing After Loss: Daily Meditations for Working Through Grief*
- Annie Kagan ~ *The Afterlife of Billy Fingers: How My Bad-Boy Brother Proved to Me There's Life After Death*
- Alexandra Kennedy ~ *Honoring Grief*
- John Lerma, MD ~ *Into the Light: Real Life Stories about Angelic Visits, Visions of the Afterlife, and Other Pre-Death Experiences*
- Anita Moorjani ~ *Dying to Be Me*
- Mary C. Neal, MD ~ *To Heaven and Back: A Doctor's Extraordinary Account of Her Death, Heaven, Angels, and Life Again: A True Story*
- Randy Pausch ~ *The Last Lecture*
- Sogyal Rinpoche ~ *Tibetan Book of Living & Dying*
- Dr. Penny Satori ~ *Wisdom of Near Death Experiences: How Understanding NDEs Can Help Us Live More Fully*
- Kathleen Dowling Singh ~ *Grace in Dying*

- Bronnie Ware ~ *Top 5 Regrets of the Dying*
- Alan D. Wolfelt, PhD ~ *Understanding Your Grief Journal*

Mind-Body; Chronic Pain

- Byron Katie ~ *Loving What Is* www.theWork.com (Recommended; audio version.)
- Robert Emmons, PhD ~ *Thanks! How Practicing Gratitude Can Make You Happier*
- Les Fehmi, PhD ~ Dissolving *Pain* (with CD) www.openfocus.com (Recommended)
- Michelle Gielan ~ *Broadcasting Happiness: The Science of Igniting and Sustaining Positive Change*
- HeartMath Institute www.heartmath.org Learn about heart variability and how it relates to stress and health; check out the emWave2. (Recommended)
- Edward Kondrot, MD ~ *Healing the Eye* www.healingtheeye.com
- Also, www.naturaleyecare.com. In addition, check out the successful Danish acupuncture systems for eyes (Dalhgren & Otte's Micro-acupuncture and Boel's Acunova); available in the US on a limited basis. Visit www.macupuncture.com for more information.
- Bruce Lipton, PhD ~ *The Biology of Belief*
- Monroe Institute ~ *Surgical Support Series*
- Nick Ortner ~ *The Tapping Solution for Pain Relief: A Step-by-Step Guide to Reducing and Eliminating Chronic Pain* www.thetappingsolution.com
- Candace Pert, PhD ~ *Molecules of Emotion*

- Positive Psychology and The Science of Happiness ~ Various resources including Rick Hanson, PhD (*Hardwiring Happiness*); Tal Ben-Shahar, Catherine Sanderson; and, www.AuthenticHappiness.sas.upenn.edu.

- Lissa Rankin, MD ~ *Mind Over Medicine* www.LissaRankin.com (Recommended)

- John Sarno, MD ~ *Healing Back Pain; The Mind-Body Prescription*

Energy Psychology & Healing; and Modern Spirituality (contemporary perspectives on ancient traditions)

- Adyashanti ~ *Falling into Grace*

- Stephen Bodian ~ *Wake Up Now*

- Gary Chapman ~ *The Five Love Languages*

- Pema Chodron ~ *Living Beautifully with Uncertainty and Change*

- Marlise Karlin ~ *The Simplicity of Stillness* www.thesosmethod.com (Recommended)

- Scott Kiloby ~ *Living Realization: A Simple, Plain-English Guide to Non-Duality* (and how to develop thought-free awareness in everyday life)

- Frank Kinslow, DC ~ *The Kinslow System: Your Path to Proven Success in Health, Love, and Life* (Classes available online at www.kinslowsystem.com.)

- Joey Klein ~ *The Inner Matrix: A Guide to Transforming Your Life and Awakening Your Spirit* www.JoeyKlein.com

RESOURCES

- Max Lucado ~ Various Christian inspired books
- Kristin Neff, PhD ~ *Self-Compassion: The Proven Power of Being Kind to Yourself* www.self-compassion.org (Recommended)
- Friar Richard Rohr ~ *Immortal Diamond; What the Mystics Know*
- Mas Sajady ~ *21-Day Medi-Healing* (online program) www.Mas-Sajady.com

Acknowledgements

No book emerges solely out of one individual's imagination. A book develops out of the coming together of countless experiences, influences, and gentle inspirations, as well as the support and assistance of others. In my case, I would be remiss not to first honor the thousands of nursing home, rehab, and ALF residents, including my parents, who have graced my path and taught me so much about life and suffering. I've also had many teachers along the way, too numerous to mention, yet each important in their own right. The lessons learned have stayed with me through the years; sometimes easing my way through life, while at other times prodding me to find deeper answers and new ways of understanding and living life.

More recently, Norman Waara (husband and first-line editor), Beth Berman, and Beverly LaRock were significant in molding this book to what it is today. A special measure of gratitude to editor extraordinaire, Elizabeth Zack (Bookcraftersllc.com). A heartfelt thank you to each and everyone, including the reader, who hopefully will gain greater peace and clarity from these words.

About the Author

Ileana Báscuas, PhD, ABPP, has been a Licensed Psychologist for over thirty-five years. "Dr. B" is also Board Certified in Clinical Psychology by the American Board of Professional Psychology. Beginning in the 1970s, Dr. B worked in children and adult services as well as mental health training and management. In 1994, Dr. B began working exclusively in nursing homes, including rehab, and assisted living facilities (ALFs) in Florida.

Dr. B has dealt with these issues as a clinician, as her father's care manager for almost five years, as the primary support for both her mother as she faded unto death and her husband with his bilateral knee replacement surgery and rehab. These personal and professional experiences pushed Dr. B to study many different ways of dealing with life's physical and emotional challenges as well as methods to cope with rehab, long-term care, and the challenges of aging. For more information and blogs, visit:

www.GettingOlderBeingHere.com.

CPSIA information can be obtained
at www.ICGtesting.com
Printed in the USA
LVHW08s1352181018
594029LV00016B/515/P